DIAGNOSED

DIAGNOSED

An Insider's Guide for Your Healthcare Journey

CRIS ROSS ✚ ED MARX

MAYO CLINIC PRESS

MAYO CLINIC PRESS
200 First St. SW
Rochester, MN 55905
mcpress.mayoclinic.org

The information in this book is true and complete to the best of our knowledge.
This book is intended as an informative guide for those wishing to learn more
about health issues. It is not intended to replace, countermand or conflict with
advice given to you by your own physician. The ultimate decision concerning
your care should be made between you and your doctor. Information in this
book is offered with no guarantees.

The author and publisher disclaim all liability in connection with the use of
this book.

The views expressed are the author's personal views, and do not necessarily
reflect the policy or position of Mayo Clinic.

To stay informed about Mayo Clinic Press, please subscribe to our free
e-newsletter at mcpress.mayoclinic.org or follow us on social media.

For bulk sales to employers, member groups and health-related companies,
contact Mayo Clinic at SpecialSalesMayoBooks@mayo.edu.

100% of author royalties from the sale of this book benefit important medical
research at Mayo Clinic Comprehensive Cancer Center.

Front cover art: bagira22/iStock via Getty Images

Library of Congress Control Number: 2023058832
Cataloging-in-Publication Data is available upon request

ISBN 979-8-88770-034-2 paperback
ISBN 979-8-88770-035-9 ebook

Printed in the United States of America
First edition: 2024

To the first woman I ever loved, my mother, Ida Wilhelmina Kollmansberger. From you I learned grace, mercy, love, and hope. Perhaps most of all, resilience. I know you are thrilled to see a book that will help people better navigate their health journey.

—Ed

To my daughters, Emily and Hannah.

—Cris

Contents

Foreword

Tia Newcomer
CEO of CaringBridge

When you or a loved one receive a difficult diagnosis, your world is turned upside down. Instantly. You are faced with a barrage of questions, decisions, emotions, and uncertainties. You may feel overwhelmed, scared, angry, or hopeless. You may wonder how to cope, how to communicate, how to navigate the complex healthcare system, and how to find the best possible care and support.

You are not alone.

Diagnosed is your essential guide as a patient or a caregiver. It empowers you to create a positive and meaningful patient experience for yourself or your loved one. Based on Ed's and Cris's personal healthcare journeys and professional insights, as well as on research and interviews with experts, caregivers, and patients from diverse backgrounds and conditions, it covers topics such as:

- How to process the shock and grief of a diagnosis and find hope and resilience.
- How to communicate effectively with your healthcare team, family, friends, and community.

- How to advocate for yourself (or, as a caregiver, for your loved one) in the healthcare system and beyond.
- How to access and use the best available resources, tools, and technologies to support your care and recovery.
- How to create a personalized care plan that reflects your values, goals, and preferences.
- How to cope with the physical, emotional, mental, social, and spiritual aspects of your health journey.
- How to celebrate your milestones, honor your losses, and embrace your new normal.

Because of my experience as the CEO of CaringBridge and my own personal journey of supporting my husband through his cancer diagnosis—twice—I am cheering as this book empowers caregivers and patients with tangible tools to address the scary, unforgiving, and overwhelming moments of a health journey.

At CaringBridge, our vision is a world in which no one goes through a health journey alone. For over 25 years, we have been providing a platform that surrounds people going through a health journey with support and connection. We have seen firsthand the power of love, hope, and compassion in healing.

Cris joined the CaringBridge board of directors between his two cancer episodes; I met him halfway through his second treatment as I became CEO. What I appreciate most about this book is the way Cris and Ed share their experiences as patients, healthcare professionals—and survivors.

Every health journey deserves a voice, a community, and a way forward. This book helps you find your voice, your community, and your way forward.

This is also a must-read resource for healthcare providers, leaders, and organizations who want to understand and improve the patient perspective and deliver patient-centered and compassionate care, inclusive of the role of the family caregiver.

Diagnosed will be on our organization's digital bookshelf of resources—for patients, caregivers, and the communities surrounding them with support. I hope you will read it and share it with others who may benefit from its wisdom and guidance. I'm proud to stand with Ed and Cris as leaders who are trying to make a difference in the lives of the millions of people facing health challenges. Support creates a better future for every patient and their loved ones. *Diagnosed* offers that support.

Part One

Voices from the Front Lines

We wrote this book while still recovering from our own healthcare battles. What you will read is unvarnished, straight from the gut. It even presents still-painful emotions that we experienced during our journeys.

This is not a book for the faint of heart or for those looking for platitudes about illness. This is as real as it gets. In fact, we had to take a pause in our writing when Cris's colorectal cancer came back with a vengeance. But as a result of our arduous healthcare battles, we are able to provide you with heartfelt insights and perspectives and, hopefully, useful tips, ideas, and tricks to ensure that you have the best health journey possible.

While we are similar in many ways, each of us approached our health journey in a different way and with a different style. You will see that in our writing. This is a good thing. There is no one right way to be an empowered patient or to maximize your health journey.

From Ed: Cris may not put it this way, but I see that Cris rolls with the punches and doesn't get very high or low. He's pretty steady. His approach is calm, responsive to circumstances, and more private than mine—even though having cancer strike him twice in rapid succession shook him to his core. I would say his approach is practical for those who like to take one step at a time with a smaller circle of support.

From Cris: Ed is more like a fighter. More direct. He has an "I will vanquish you before you vanquish me" kind of persona. Given his army training and experience, he is big on strategy and planning. His approach is super-practical for those who like to write things out, and he plots each healthcare move with conscious intent. He also gathers groups of folks around him because of his outgoing, loving nature, and as a result, he receives great love and support from them.

You may find yourself gravitating toward one of our approaches more than the other, or you may find you are comfortable somewhere in between the two. You will probably discover that sometimes it is preferable to be super-detailed in your planning, but you may also feel that too much structure adds more stress. Or you might discover that for you, a freestyle "go with the flow" approach leads to a feeling of loss of control.

Many patients in our focus groups adopted different styles at different stages of their journey, depending on specific circumstances at specific times. A structured approach may be helpful early on, while there are many choices to make, but then as the journey intensifies maintaining a more agile posture may work best. You will figure out the approach or combination of approaches for you. You do you.

We are here to show you your choices and offer you help in making them.

Consider this book a hand you can hold on your journey.

With love and respect,
Ed Marx and Cris Ross

One

So You've Been Diagnosed

So you've been diagnosed with a challenging medical condition. Or maybe you have a family member or friend who is ill and needs your support. We're truly sorry. We've been through our own journeys and have supported family and friends on theirs. We have experienced the feelings and challenges you are facing. You are not alone in your journey. We will walk you through this.

Why We Wrote This Book

This book is a how-to guide for patients, family, and friends to create a best-possible patient experience throughout a challenging healthcare journey. We get you. We have been there—the shock, the fear, the loneliness, the anger. And we know that you are dealing with the emotions of a challenging diagnosis, as well as wondering how you are going to navigate a healthcare system that is confusing and frustrating. We want to help with both. As former patients, we want to share our journeys to help you with yours. As healthcare executives, we want to give you our insider's view of how healthcare works and how you can navigate it.

IF YOU NEED A QUICK START

We recognize that sometimes you want advice pronto on how to cope with a serious diagnosis—no time to read a whole book before you set out to get the best care possible. So, for any of you who find yourselves in a time crunch, having to make immediate decisions about your care, we have included a **Quick Start Guide** later in this chapter.

We wish this book weren't necessary. Yet, as we learned the hard way, nothing in our service as healthcare executives in the world's foremost hospitals adequately prepared us, or our families and friends, for this journey. We wish we'd had a book like this to help us during our health crises.

But there was no book available that gave us the guidance we were looking for. No how-to guide that helped us handle some of the hardest moments of our lives. We knew that if we, as industry insiders, struggled, those with little experience would face even more difficulties trying to navigate the complexities of our healthcare system. So we wrote the book we wish we'd had then.

Even though we're sharing the knowledge and ideas contained in this book, we can't promise you smooth sailing. We will give you some tools to create your own best journey, and some ideas that have the potential to improve your health outcome. You may find some of our ideas too simplistic and others too complex. Some of the homework you may not find doable, while sometimes you might want more. We encourage you to use this book as a guide. You can do much of what we suggest, or you can just take on pieces and parts.

So Who Are We?

We are two healthcare executives who had significant medical journeys. Ed was the chief information officer at Cleveland Clinic and now runs his own healthcare technology advisory company. Cris is the chief information officer at Mayo Clinic. Ed had a near-fatal heart attack and prostate cancer, and Cris had to contend with two rounds of stage 3 colorectal cancer.

> *Ed: I have been—and continue to be—a serious athlete committed to wellness. So you can imagine how it upended my world to first have a heart attack and then develop cancer. I had to rethink who I was and my place on the earth. And because I was blessed with good outcomes from both, I can say that I came out the other side humbled, overwhelmed with my love for family and friends, and ferociously committed to helping everyone who has to find their way as they deal with doctors and hospitals.*

> *Cris: Finding the internal strength—twice—to face advanced colorectal cancer was an illuminating process, and one I could not have gone through without the support of family and friends, as well as a willingness to stand up to my care team when I knew in my heart that what I wanted was right for me. That wasn't easy for me, but it taught me something I want to share with other people contending with potentially life-altering medical decisions.*

We learned firsthand that the patient experience is not what it should be even at two of the world's most elite healthcare organizations (Cleveland Clinic and Mayo Clinic). We also learned that the best possible patient experience when dealing with an aspirational but imperfect healthcare system fundamentally depends on how you, the patient, approach your journey.

We acknowledge that we write from positions of significant privilege. We are both white, male, and born in the 1960s. We are well-educated and have successful careers. We have been married, have adult children, and have active social lives. We understand we are not representative of everyone. We have worked hard to avoid developing a framework that only works for people who look or live like us.

As you go through the book, you will meet a variety of people who share their healthcare journey with you. There's Debra, a Native American, who battled to have her hypertrophic cardiomyopathy diagnosed; Mark, who ran into almost every obstacle to quality care imaginable and emerged triumphant; Ginger, a woman with multiple health challenges, who fought to find empathy in her care team; Amelia, who struggled to find caring, knowledgeable treatment as she transitioned; and Deb, who finally found compassionate doctors who worked with and for her to find solutions to her severe asthma. You'll also hear from some of our caregivers, pulling back the curtain on how they coped in the most private of moments.

So, are you ready to get started?

∾

QUICK START: YOU ARE IN THE MIDDLE OF THE MUDDLE

Medical Emergencies

Someone with a medical emergency won't have time to pick up this book. This book is not really aimed at helping you navigate the emergency department. But if you are ever in that situation or are advising a family member or friend, with little time or few choices of doctors or hospitals, or you are in a rural environment without a lot of options, a few things are key. It is important that:

- All information about your prior medical diagnoses and prescriptions is known to your medical caregivers.
- Your diagnosis and symptoms are explained clearly to you and/or someone who is there with you.
- You ask for as much information as possible.
- You have someone to help you remember, help you understand what you're hearing, and even make decisions for you if you are unable to manage your situation. This is very important—even vital.

Fortunately, emergency departments are well equipped and trained to deal with these situations.

Essential Questions and Information to Share

Whether you have a troubling symptom and want your primary care doctor to help, or you have been referred to a specialist, asking the doctors you interact with the following questions will help you understand what is happening, increase your ability to participate in treatment decisions, and improve your patient experience.

1. What is my diagnosis? What is that based on? Who made the diagnosis?

2. Who is the doctor in charge of my case?
3. What kind of specialist should I be treated by—and when can that person see me?
4. Can you contact and work with my primary care doctor? Can all my medical records be shared?
5. Do you have an accurate list of all the medications and supplements I am taking, and can we go over the list together?
6. What are the pros and cons of the recommended treatments? Are there alternatives?
7. Do I need to decide immediately what treatment I will receive, or can I take some time to do research before I decide?
8. *If applicable:* Who in each medical office and hospital needs to know the name of my healthcare proxy and the name of the person who has my medical power of attorney?
9. If I want, can I be transferred from this facility to another of my choice? How do I arrange that?
10. What do you typically recommend for people in my situation and how much experience do you and/or the physicians you are referring me to have treating my condition?
11. *If you are heading into surgery:* Who is performing the surgery? What are their credentials and experience? How many of these surgeries have they done?
12. Do you accept my insurance? Will the doctors who see me and the services I receive be covered? What will my out-of-pocket expenses be?

Ideally, write down the answers to these questions so that you will remember them later. If it's not possible for you to write them down, see if someone might be willing to help you take notes. You can also try using your phone to make notes about what is said. Do whatever you can to retain the information. Your mind will be going in many different directions, and remembering everything that's said will be challenging.

You Have the Right to Choose

Remember, in all but the most extreme circumstances you have a choice of doctors and hospitals. If you were ordering a pizza, you'd look up reviews on Yelp. If you were buying a car, you'd check various auto magazines and consumer guides. When it comes to medical care, you should choose doctors and hospitals with at least the same rigor that you'd use in picking a restaurant or buying a car. For example, if you are told you need surgery but the surgery can wait, insist on finding out about other options, and choose the surgeon who is best for you and your particular medical needs.

Next Steps

Think about you—what will give you resilience, strength, and hope. In an urgent medical situation, once you have been diagnosed and first treatments have been administered, you're then facing future treatments, recovery, the unknown. You want to take steps to improve your experience.

A key step in optimizing the situation is to nurture and build resilience. It's an ongoing process. If you are in a rushed medical situation, you can't say, "Wait, I'm going to build some resilience and then we can begin treatment." You have to build it along the way.

Consider the following five proven ways to build resilience. Which are most powerful for you? Which ones will help you get through the next days and weeks?

- Be proactive. What needs to be done? Make plans and take action.
- Take care of yourself. Be as good to yourself as you would be to a loved one under these circumstances. You matter.
- Learn from experience. How have you coped with hardship in the past?

- Get connected. Depend on and build relationships.
- Make every day meaningful. Set achievable goals while focusing on the future.

Remember, although you are not better informed than your doctor about medical matters, you are the expert on you. The clearer you are about your intentions, wishes, fears, and questions, the better your journey will be.

Begin to gather your friends and family around you. Identify who can offer assistance and support as you go through your patient experience. Some folks can be at your bedside when you're in the hospital. Some can feed your pets and water your plants. Others can be a warm voice on the phone. And some will participate with or for you in making medical decisions.

Never stop asking questions. You have every right to know about your care, your care team, and the treatments you are being given—or not being given.

Fight for your health and happiness in whatever way suits you, but remember that you want your healthcare providers to be on your team. So you need to recognize that they are people too and deserve respect and patience, as well as thanks and gratitude for what they are doing for you. Join forces whenever possible.

Exploring the Book

Once you've been diagnosed and things settle down, you'll have some time to gather your wits and make a plan. We have created a framework aimed at improving your healthcare experience going forward.

Health journeys can be confusing and scary, so we created a visual that might serve as a map. There are five components to our patient experience model. We will define them below and then explore each of them more fully in subsequent chapters.

How We Developed the Framework

First, we researched the academic and industry literature on the patient experience. Thankfully, many people are studying how patients feel when they talk to their doctors or get information on their health condition. Healthcare workers are trying to figure out where the problems are in their systems and make improvements to help people interact better with all the hospital staff they encounter, from medical assistants to surgeons; to address how respected or neglected patients might feel; and to find ways to upgrade the hospital experience (for example, whether the food could be better, whether the halls are too noisy, and whether the rooms are sufficiently comfortable).

We also interviewed respected leaders on resiliency, empathy, and experience. We were purposeful in reaching out to hundreds of people in and outside of healthcare. We coordinated and led dozens of focus groups, incorporating participants' feedback and insights. We tested our framework with members of still-marginalized communities. We met with persons from many backgrounds to ensure that our ideas are practical for most. The book also strives to include experiences and perspectives that define us, Ed and Cris, as individuals.

Then, based on our own experience as patients and as executives with industry insights, we developed a model for how you can improve your interactions and outcomes as you strive to reclaim your best possible health.

We are aware of the limits of our experience and knowledge. Our experience is with cancer, a heart attack, and caring for our families. Neither of us pretends to know from our lived experience what it's like to need an organ transplant, manage a long-term chronic or debilitating condition, or receive care in a small or challenged hospital or a public-access clinic reimbursed by Medicaid. That's why we say that our model is not the only model but describes what we experienced as patients and observed as insiders. We hope it provides a decent framework for how to play the health cards you've been dealt.

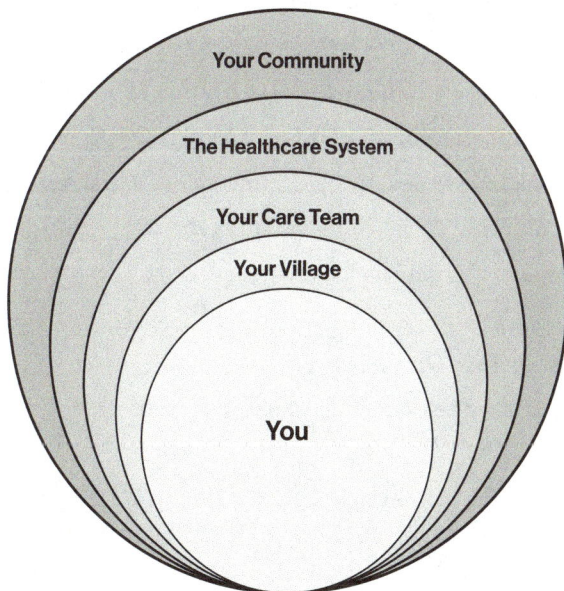

We would encourage you to go into some depth on each ring of the framework, but again, this is completely up to you. You are free to use the entirety of the framework or perhaps just aspects of it. Whatever works for you. Whatever makes you comfortable.

You and Your Journey

We'd Like You to Meet Yourself

The center of a serious healthcare journey is you, the person with the challenging diagnosis. Despite the fact that there are millions of people and millions of unique journeys toward health, we believe there is one truth for all patients: the best possible interaction with the healthcare system begins with *you*, the patient, being clear with yourself and others about your intentions for the journey.

We agree with studies that show that a patient's attitudes can affect quality of life throughout a healthcare journey. As our attitudes shifted through our months of care, we developed a nonscientific but strongly held opinion that your approach and attitude as you go through a serious healthcare journey need to be true to yourself. It's easy to get overwhelmed and swept away by the intensity of a healthcare journey, but we think being anchored in the self is the key to everything else. We will explore this more in Chapter 4.

Participate in Your Own Journey

Sometimes a story helps in understanding an idea.

> *Ed: Some time ago, my coworkers and I embarked on a weekend trip to raft the Youghiogheny River.*

Because it was my first rafting experience, I listened keenly to the instructors explaining how to navigate the river and what to do in the event the raft flips or you otherwise fall overboard. "Participate in your own rescue!" they shouted over and over as they explained survival techniques.

They taught us to do the following if we fell into the water.

1. *If the guide can't get to you from another raft, keep your legs up and point them downstream.*
2. *If the rescue kayak does not reach you, stay focused. Keep your legs up and facing downstream, and keep your head up.*
3. *In the most dangerous sections, one of the staff is on top of a boulder in the middle of the river. Listen to her instructions.*
4. *But no matter what, participate in your own rescue.*

I was the first to fall out.

I turned to focus on the woman atop the boulder. She threw her rope across the path I was most likely to take on the now raging river. "Participate in my own rescue," I said to myself over and over.

I caught the rope in front of me and held on for dear life as I hit the eddies and tumbled underwater like a shirt in the washing machine. I could not give up. I could not count on anyone to rescue me. I had to participate in my own rescue.

I emerged from the eddies as the woman pulled me to safety. I've never rafted again, but I learned the lesson the river had for me.

If there is a single lesson in this book, it is this: participate in your journey.

Nobody can take your place. Nobody can walk this journey for you. But even though that is 100 percent true, you don't have to be alone.

Don't Go It Alone

The second big lesson in this book is how to assemble a village of people around you and a care team that you can depend upon. Doing that successfully is contingent on how fully you initially—and continuously—participate in your own journey. Because we've been through this too, we seek to be your fellow travelers. You are why we wrote this book. Let's do this together.

Ideally, a Village

When faced with a health crisis, there can be a temptation to retreat from others and hold everything in. It's easy to become so stressed and burdened that you withdraw from friends and family. While this can be a natural—and in some ways important—coping reaction, it is vital to resist becoming isolated or lonely.

As the saying goes, it takes a village. So we hope you have a community of family and friends who are there to support you. We also know this is not always the case. For those of you with a strong village of family and/or friends, consider yourself lucky and read through for ideas that might make your village stronger. If family and/or friends are sparse, we share some ideas on how to create a village that might be just you and a caregiver, and how you might grow or create your village in unlikely ways. You can and should reach out to others and have the courage and humility to accept help when it is offered.

For those of you with family and friends who are willing to help, there are some things to become aware of. For example, family and friends have their own feelings and worries about something like a cancer diagnosis. Some may think, *Will my loved one die?* Others may worry, *What am I supposed to say and do?* Or, *Someone close to me died from cancer, and I can't face this again.* And some may think, *My loved one isn't approaching their care correctly and should have a different attitude!*

Also, village members may not be sure how to help. Like patients, members of a village have their own contexts and experiences, which they bring to their interactions with "their" patient's health journey. Some village members may even need to be kept at arm's length.

This book was written by two guys with very different approaches to building a village. We know from comparing our experiences that there is no one best way. There are different ways to safely reach out to others. We provide some diverse ideas about how to give yourself permission to ask for help, and how to let those around you know what you need and what they can do.

Building Your Care Team

When you are diagnosed and then go into the hospital, you will discover that there are a lot of people assigned to take care of you in one way or another. We call these people—the doctors, specialists, nurses, assistants, doctor's office staff members, people pushing you around on a bed—your care team.

In short, your care team is made up of everyone who delivers medical and custodial care or makes decisions about what kinds of care are available and delivered. Some of these people you will interact with directly at one time or another. Some are part of the "invisible" staff in the hospital or clinic who help with and sometimes guide your care.

The first duty of the medical members of your care team is to create a treatment plan and define the path and milestones for care. They are the ones who provide answers to the following questions:

- What is the diagnosis and prognosis?
- What are the options for treatment and care?
- What should the patient expect?
- What actions can the patient take to improve their odds of successful and easy treatment?
- How can care providers take a patient's priorities and preferences into account?

In Chapter 4 we write about the choices you can make to ensure you have the right care team, are comfortable with them, and know how to engage with them. Ideally, you, your village, and your care team will be aligned in your journey.

Learning to Interact with Your Care Team

Especially when you're facing a difficult diagnosis, it's natural to defer to a white-coated healthcare provider who you hope will have all the answers and perform miracles. While our clinician colleagues have our respect, have answers to almost everything, and often do seemingly miraculous things, the best approach is to think of the patient-doctor relationship as a partnership. Deference to a care team, taken to an extreme, can create an unintentional and unhealthy relationship in which neither the patient nor the members of the patient's village have the confidence to ask questions, express preferences, or clarify recommendations. We provide practical examples of how to maintain a good balance between respect for professional expertise and self-advocacy.

The Big Issues and Annoying Things About "the System"

Your care team exists within a larger system. Patients sometimes encounter this behind-the-scenes system. It is composed of the insurance companies and government agencies that pay for care; the manufacturers of drugs, devices, and imaging tools; the researchers who find new cures and therapies; the experts at the hospitals and professional associations who define best practices for care; and so on. Sometimes the system is helpful, supportive, and easy to deal with; sometimes it is maddening and frustrating. We will cover the most common frustrations and share some insights that may help make some sense of the quagmire.

The Larger Community

It's also important to realize that the system operates in a community that establishes standards and norms by which healthcare is delivered and regulated. This can vary from country to country or in some instances from region to region. The community can have a very positive effect, such as the protection of patient privacy and confidentiality. It can also have a negative effect, particularly in the form of health inequities, in which people from different backgrounds receive different care for reasons unrelated to their diagnosis and prognosis. In some states, for example, state regulations do not support equal delivery of care to women or to transgender individuals. Having a basic knowledge of the community in which your care is delivered is helpful in gaining a better understanding of how your care may be affected and of the complicated nature of healthcare in the United States.

Connecting the Circles

These circles—your self, your village, your care team, the system, and your community—are all nested. For someone on a difficult health journey, the broader healthcare system or the community may seem remote, until it is not: when an insurer declines to pay for a particular treatment, when deductibles become overwhelming, when a desired experimental treatment is out of reach or not approved for use, and so on. Conversely, it may seem like the self and the village are insignificant, until they are not: when an individual patient is determined to pursue a particular course of treatment that does not align with the norms of the care team or system, or when the collective voice of the self and the village advocates for change to a system or community that is not responsive to the needs of patients.

In the healthcare environment we aspire to, all these circles are nested. The patient has a strong and clear sense of self and can express their intentions for care. Those intentions are heard by the care team and supported by the village. The system is malleable enough to support a variety of patient intentions and pathways, and it provides support rather than erecting barriers. The community is both empathetic and scientific, it provides equal opportunity for those moving through the system, and it establishes guardrails so that inadequacies are remedied.

We know that this is an aspiration rather than a description of what we have today. Despite remarkable progress and places of distinguished achievement, as a whole the American healthcare system is imperfect and can do better. So while this book is intended to help you with your journey, you may find that you too want to make things better for the next person. If so, come join us as we advocate for the healthcare we want.

How to Use This Book

It is our hope that this framework for patient experience provides tools you can use to help navigate your healthcare journey. The chapters on self (Chapter 4), village (Chapter 5), and care team (Chapter 6) have action items we encourage you to follow. They contain ideas you can use to make your journey or that of your loved one more manageable. The action items will help you create a guide that provides specific direction for you, your village, and your care team.

In the next two chapters, we will describe our healthcare experiences as a way of walking with you. This is your journey and your journey only, but you are not alone.

Two

Inside Out

Cris Ross's journey from healthcare
exec to patient—and back again

In early 2018, Mayo Clinic was approaching the most critical stage in the most challenging and risky project I'd ever encountered in my career.

On May 5, we were poised to replace virtually all our technology for medical care and billing at our Rochester, Minnesota, flagship location. In a hospital, everything depends on technology: diagnosis, documentation, treatment, communication with patients, medical devices, billing—everything. We were going to change almost all of it, all at once. A lot was on the line. Our then-CEO called this the biggest project in our 160-year history. But as we approached the big date, I was miserable.

In my teens through my early thirties, I wrestled with what today might be diagnosed as irritable bowel syndrome. I had become accustomed to constant gut aches and interruptions to daily life. But now, twenty years later, it seemed to have returned at the worst possible time—I had a huge amount of work to do. I chalked it up to the stress of the project, pressed through it, and committed to getting checked out right after we finished the big technology change.

By early July our mega-project had stabilized. At this point discomfort had changed to real pain. I noticed blood in my stool for the first time. I got in as soon as I could with my primary care doctor, Joanna Rea, on Monday, July 16. By then I was convinced this wasn't just irritable bowel syndrome but something seriously wrong. Mayo moves quickly. Two days later, on Wednesday, July 18, I had a colonoscopy. On Thursday, July 19, I had a CT scan and pathology results from colonoscopy samples.

A Cancer Diagnosis

The same day as my CT scan I walked over to Dr. Rea's office in an adjacent clinic building, where I was joined by my girlfriend, Anne-Marie, a radiologist at Mayo. We received the news together. "I'm sorry," said Dr. Rea. "You have colorectal cancer."

As a chief information officer, I'm used to bad news—it's not uncommon for me to deal with several real or imagined emergencies per day. Our giant project had had me on high alert for months. My immediate response to this cancer diagnosis was not to be sad or afraid but to treat it as just another big and complex problem that needed to be solved: this cancer needs to be cured, so let's get on with it. It didn't feel personal yet, but it did feel urgent.

I asked many questions: Whom could I talk with? What were the options? What would treatment look like? How could I evaluate this problem, find root causes, make corrections, and move through it successfully? How could I keep my professional and personal life going while attending to this emergency?

Appointments were scheduled with gastroenterology, oncology, and surgery. I had an MRI scan of my pelvis on Friday, July 20, the day after receiving my diagnosis. Over the weekend I reached out to many colleagues for advice. All were generous with their time and empathy. I learned that my situation had already been discussed on Friday by a "tumor board," an interdisciplinary group of doctors. On Monday, July 23, I met the oncologist assigned to my case, Dr. Thor Halfdanarson, and radiation oncologist Dr. Michael Haddock. Thor told me that my cancer was stage 3, which is pretty bad. It was a large tumor, but luckily it had not spread elsewhere in my body. (When a cancer has spread to other parts of the body, it is called metastatic cancer; that is stage 4 cancer and can be very hard to cure.) At this meeting Thor said the clinical intent was to cure me of cancer. This surprised me, and I asked, "Don't you intend to cure everyone?" He gently and carefully explained that while some cancers can be cured, others can only be contained. On Tuesday, July 24, I met with my assigned surgeon, Dr. Scott Kelley. On July 27, eleven days after my first consultation with my primary care physician, I had a port placed in my chest and received my first dose of chemotherapy.

My recollection of those eleven days is both crystal clear and a blur. As Ed and I will explore in other chapters, different people respond differently to these kinds of health crises. We believe the only "correct" response is the one that is authentic to you, the person receiving the diagnosis, and to the people closest to you.

My way of responding to this serious diagnosis was pretty simple. First, I wanted to be honest with my family and friends. Anne-Marie had accompanied me to my appointments and was fully informed. I talked via video with my older daughter, Hannah, in Seattle. I sat down with my younger daughter, Emily, who was living with me in St. Paul after recently returning from four years living in Paris. Both took the news quietly and calmly, asked a few questions, were scared, and offered support. I told everyone close to me what I understood as the truth: I had a tumor that was serious but curable. I intended to beat it. I would answer their questions as best I could. I honestly did not feel afraid, perhaps because I was too ignorant to know what to be afraid of, but also because I had seen what Mayo Clinic could do. I believed fully that if I could simply submit to it and persevere through it, I would be cured.

The plan was laid out for me by my doctors, Thor, Michael, and Scott. They would attack the tumor with chemotherapy and radiation therapy to reduce its size and prevent spread, followed by surgery to remove the remaining cancer. I prepared for eight biweekly chemotherapy sessions, radiation therapy sessions for twenty-five consecutive days, and surgery. I took medical leave and in the interim turned over my job to my colleague and friend Mike Ryan.

I don't know whether it was because of my CIO "take action and solve this problem" stance or from some other source, but I was determined not to let cancer beat me physically, mentally, or emotionally. I wanted to step into my role as a cancer patient with integrity and purpose.

I looked around for models. A good friend, Allyson, had a daughter who had been treated twice for leukemia, once as a toddler and then as a kindergartner. Their journey was awful, but both mother and daughter emerged stronger, and each was transformed. Allyson told me she had found the "gift of cancer." She didn't choose for her daughter to have cancer; all she could do was choose how to respond to it. Her approach was to look for what the cancer journey would teach her and how she might become transformed by going through it.

So I entered cancer treatment seeking two "gifts." The first came from the intensity that goes along with my day job. I figured I had an unparalleled opportunity to see Mayo Clinic as a patient from the inside out, including the good, the bad, and the ugly of the comprehensive new software we had just launched. I sought the gift of being a better CIO when I emerged.

Second, I was determined to see how cancer could teach me to truly live life with joy and intention. I meant to keep this aspiration through treatment and survival. Cancer was unwelcome, but I didn't want it to define me. I wanted to appreciate everything I could, for as long and deeply as I could, through my cancer journey and beyond.

Becoming a Cancer Patient

With my work assignments passed to others, and my heart and head as clear as I could make them, I stepped into being a cancer patient. I was ready.

The first step was chemotherapy. It's a powerful treatment that I hope we can someday make obsolete with other therapies. It is unpleasant. But, true to my desire to learn from my cancer, I sought to learn how chemotherapy had been invented. In World War I, when poisonous mustard gas was used in battle, bone marrow and lymph nodes were depleted in men exposed to the gas. Researchers tried to determine if nitrogen mustard gas variants could treat cancers by killing cancer cells but not people. More than two decades later, research carried out prior to World War II led to additional chemotherapies. Just after the war, Babe Ruth was an early chemotherapy patient, though his cancer was too advanced, and his treatment was unsuccessful.

New forms of chemotherapy have emerged since then, but a nitrogen mustard variant is still used as part of a multidrug chemotherapy for Hodgkin lymphoma.

Different chemotherapies have different names. Mine was called FOLFOX, which is a combination of folinic acid (FOL), fluorouracil (F), and oxaliplatin (OX). A different but widely used chemotherapy for adult and childhood cancers, doxorubicin, is nicknamed "Red Devil."

Here's how it worked. Every two weeks I checked into an outpatient infusion center, where one of the amazingly empathetic and capable nurses would insert a special needle into my port, a small rubbery bulb that had earlier been inserted surgically under the skin in my chest. They taped the needle and tubes to my chest, always apologizing for how the tape would rip out hair when it was removed. I was hooked up to bags containing cocktails of chemotherapy and anti-nausea drugs that over the course of about two and a half hours were pumped through the port into a vein leading directly into my heart.

When the bags were empty, they gave me a small green satchel into which they put a new bag of drugs and a little pump, which they connected to my chest tubes. I would drive myself home with the bag over my shoulder and receive an ongoing dose for the next day and a half. Mostly I just felt sick for three to five days. The drugs made food taste weird and awful. I was tired, but sleep was sometimes hard. When the bag was empty, I would don a mask and medical gloves, disconnect the tubes, inject drugs to prevent blood clots into my port tubing, peel off the tape on my chest, and pull the needle out of the port. Anne-Marie did it for me the first time and taught me how to do it for myself. It was always satisfying to wrap up and throw away all the leftovers of chemotherapy and wash away the taste and smell with a long shower. Then I'd get down to the business of recovering from the chemo.

I had two weeks between chemo sessions and could function pretty well in my off weeks. I could exercise, do things that were enjoyable, be optimistic, and envision life beyond cancer. On one particularly memorable good weekend, my daughter Emily and I made a pilgrimage to a favorite place—the virgin forest and headwaters of the Mississippi River. We hiked, canoed, and read books around the fireplace on a rainy day. It was really easy to forget cancer that weekend. Sometimes joy came easily.

I visited Thor every other week before my chemotherapy. After four sessions another MRI showed the tumor was staying the same size or perhaps shrinking. We discussed side effects from chemo and made plans for radiation therapy and surgery.

(A side note: No one wants an oncologist, but if you need one, you want yours to be named Thor. Perhaps he has demigod powers—a guy from Iceland with rugged good looks, a world expert in the treatment of colorectal cancer, but also a very patient listener. I never felt hurried or unheard.)

I also focused on my intention to be a better CIO because of my health journey. While undergoing chemotherapy I tried to be attentive to what was working for nurses and what was not. I saw one nurse struggling to scan the plastic chemotherapy bags and learned from her that they were too shiny to be scanned easily. Scanning the bags also set a time stamp for the start of chemotherapy, which could sometimes be incorrect. I asked a lot of questions. I reported these minor but important defects to the technology team, and the issues were addressed pretty quickly. After that, I didn't need to ask in order to hear requests and gripes from the chemotherapy nurses—I tried to stay anonymous, but they quickly figured out I could help them. I was inspired to help as I sometimes cringed watching a clinician struggle with something that should have been easier to understand and use.

After eight sessions of chemotherapy over the course of sixteen weeks, I graduated to radiation therapy. To ensure that the dose was delivered to the precise location every session, I received two tiny calibration tattoos on my hips that were used to align me with laser guides on the radiation therapy machine. (The two little tats are permanent, but I remain very uncool.) A custom-fitted brace held my legs in place. For the following five weeks, Monday through Friday, I reported to radiation oncology with instructions to drink enough water so that my bladder would be completely full, pressing the small intestine out of the pelvis and away from the field of radiation. I would step into a cubicle, strip to my underwear, put on a gown, and wait my turn. I was grateful to be treated with respect, because I felt vulnerable, cold, exposed, and sometimes more like a medical object than a person. When I was called, I would hop on a table, where the radiation techs would position me perfectly, and I'd lie as still as I could for about fifteen minutes (with a very full bladder) as a photon-spewing arm moved over and around my abdomen. As I lay still, I visualized a stream of photons smashing at the speed of light into the tumor, blasting and killing tumor cells.

At least for me, radiation therapy at first was relatively benign, almost undetectable. Near the end of treatment, the tumor on my colon became scarred and damaged, and that caused problems with the way my colon functioned (an unpleasant harbinger of things to come).

When radiation therapy is complete, it's traditional to ring a ship's bell in the waiting area outside radiation treatment areas. It gives hope to all of us enduring the journey. On December 21, 2018, I rang the bell with Hannah, Emily, and Anne-Marie. I was grateful that, in addition to everything else, Dr. Haddock had helped schedule things so that I could finish up my therapy before Christmas. Though I was seeking to live with joy, and at many points during my journey my treatment care team did everything they could to make that possible, I sometimes felt the joy was thrust upon me—even when it was ultimately gratifying.

With chemo and radiation done, I had a gap in treatment. From January through mid-March 2019, I had a period of relative normalcy. I returned to work on a couple of special projects—more for my sake than Mayo's. The most important during this period was creating a milestone agreement with Google to apply advanced data and artificial intelligence to medical care. One of our initial projects was the use of artificial intelligence to improve planning of radiation therapy. I also had an opportunity to speak from the heart at a large industry conference to an audience of thousands, describing my journey through cancer.

The final stage of my journey was surgery to remove my rectum and the tumor that had invaded it, scheduled for March 13, 2019. Before this diagnosis, I had never had surgery, nor had I spent a night in a hospital except as a support when my children were born. I was anxious, so just before surgery I visited my daughter Hannah in Seattle to take my mind off things. We did normal things we like to do together—see weird theater, try new bars, eat street food, and visit historical sites. For me, getting away was the perfect preparation for surgery—more joy and distraction. I think it helped Hannah to see me pretty healthy, laughing and talking about things we both like. I returned to Minnesota and with Anne-Marie's help reported for surgery at 5:30 a.m. on March 13, my anxiety much lower because I had distracted myself by visiting Hannah and spending the evening before surgery with Anne-Marie.

Surgical prep, at least at Mayo Clinic, is careful, scripted, and remarkably quiet and unhurried. I was gowned, my consent and advance directives were reviewed, and pre-surgical medications were administered. The nurses were calm and empathetic as I sat in a hospital bed in the pre-op area. When my time came, I was rolled through the hallways to operating room 83 in Rochester Methodist Hospital.

My surgeon, Scott Kelley, inspires immediate confidence. He has a boyish fighter-pilot demeanor that isn't uncommon among surgeons. As I lay on the table mostly naked in a cooled operating suite, staring up at acoustic tiles, lights, and ceiling-mounted surgical equipment, he knew exactly when and how to put his hand on my shoulder and tell me they were going to take good care of me.

I woke up in the perioperative recovery area, with no sense of the passage of time, though I had been in surgery for about seven hours. I knew I would have a temporary ostomy to reroute the contents of my intestines through a surgical opening in my abdomen into a removable bag on my belly. I would need that for several weeks while my intestines healed. I reached down to feel the bag. I also became aware of inflatable booties rhythmically squeezing my feet to reduce the risk of blood clots. From the recovery room, I was rolled to an elevator and up to my hospital room. I felt alert pretty quickly, but definitely beat up. I met the nursing team, who told me I needed to stand and go for a short walk.

As I mentioned, this was my first surgery. I had a freshly closed incision from sternum to pubic bone with a bag hanging from my belly. I found it nearly inconceivable that I could be walking a few hours after being wide open on a surgical table. But I was in no position to object. With nursing help, I used a walker-type device to shuffle a hundred feet or so. I was also surprised at how little pain I felt.

The following morning the surgical team made rounds. One of the best practices at Mayo Clinic is that samples of diseased tissues are evaluated by pathologists during surgery so that a surgeon knows whether they have fully removed a tumor with clean margins. With that information, the surgeons can either continue the surgery to remove additional diseased tissue or conclude the surgery with confidence that all the cancerous tissue has been safely removed. This helps avoid the need for additional surgery later if positive pathology results are returned after the first procedure. In my case, Scott reported that my tumor had responded "phenomenally" to the chemo and radiation therapy, with lots of dead tumor tissue. There were wide clean margins around the tumor tissue that was removed. Anne-Marie and Emily were with me to hear the news as I was declared cancer-free on March 14, 2019.

Now my attention turned to healing. I tried to walk the hospital floors as if I were training for a marathon, and I sought to return to a seminormal diet. Unfortunately, my body disagreed with me on day three of recovery, and I developed ileus—a condition in which the intestines stop functioning properly. That morning my bout of *Exorcist*-class vomiting seemed to surprise even the veteran nurse who was caring for me, who I thought had seen everything. A planned five-day hospital stay extended to 10 as my condition eventually stabilized and normalized.

By the end of my stay, I really wanted to go home. I had been declared cancer-free, and I wanted to rush back to my regular life. I returned to work three weeks after my discharge from surgery. Six weeks after my first surgery, I had a second surgery to remove the temporary ostomy, which Scott referred to as "the friend you don't want but need." After a few days in the hospital recovering from the second surgery, I went home again. The post-surgery period was mostly unremarkable. At one point the incision from my second surgery became infected, and I got pretty sick and spent a night in the ER. The next day the nursing team reopened the incision and taught me how to clean and pack the wound with gauze until it slowly healed and closed up again after a few weeks. But that didn't stop me from traveling a few weeks later to a healthcare conference in Helsinki (where I had a minor incident and got to sample medical care in Finland).

No Longer a Patient

And then . . . all the medical activity ended. I had been in an intensive 289-day struggle to get through treatment that was sometimes difficult and frightening. At my last visit I was given literature to read and some nursing instructions. I had a few follow-up appointments scheduled over the next several months, but mostly I felt like I was on my own. The team moved on to other patients, all walking the same path through the dark woods from which I had just emerged. Perhaps this experience is similar to that of soldiers dropped back abruptly into civilian life after wartime.

Health systems are getting better about creating things like "digital front doors," to make the care-seeking experience better for patients, but I think few are equally competent at creating "digital back doors"—that is, providing guidance, support, and information to people recovering from significant treatment, like me and my fellow cancer survivors. For patients like me, the experience of immediate decompression was somewhat jarring. We health system executives can do better, and we patients can do more to take care of ourselves while healthcare systems get better at this. More to come about this in Chapter 8, on the mysteries of the healthcare system and how to understand and deal with them.

Taking one step at a time, I regained strength, and my scar faded to a thin white line. I had a life that felt pretty normal, with the only real damages being loss of feeling in my hands and feet from chemotherapy-induced neuropathy (the drugs can damage nerve fibers there) and a digestive system that wasn't quite the same as before. I returned to life, to work, to joy.

As a cancer survivor, I was on a surveillance program to receive a colonoscopy every year and a CT scan of my chest and pelvis every six months to look for the return of cancer. I had clear scopes and scans in February and August 2020.

Cancer 2.0

In January 2021, I had some odd pelvic pain. Something seemed wrong. I contacted Thor to see if we could accelerate my next colonoscopy and CT scan. In late January my colonoscopy was clear, but there was a suspicious spot in my pelvis that needed to be checked out. I had a full-body PET (positron emission tomography) scan, which is incredibly sensitive at detecting cancerous tissue. A few days later I had a needle biopsy of the small suspicious mass in my pelvis.

On February 10, 2021, 699 days after I'd been declared cancer-free, Thor told me I had cancer again.

Damn.

Scans showed a tumor, a little smaller than a ping-pong ball, growing on the outer wall of my colon, tucked into my left pelvis. I was going to have to do it all over again.

Ed and I had set the intention to write this book in late 2020. I remember calling him to say our book just got more interesting because I had cancer again.

Among other things, it was time to set new goals for this journey. The goals I had established and the gifts I'd sought during my first cancer journey were very inward-focused—how to be better at my job, and how to use this experience to remind me of the importance of living with joy. I really don't have regrets about looking for those gifts, and they were still resonant for me as I began my second journey. Maybe it's because now I had creeping doubts about my mortality, or maybe it's because I gained an ability to live outside myself a little bit more, but through my second cancer journey I really felt called to use my experience to make other people's serious health journeys a little easier.

I was thinking about these intentions as my second journey through cancer began. First, I learned pretty quickly that if it was a privilege to be treated for cancer at Mayo Clinic once, the second time was an even greater privilege. Recurrent rectal cancers are really challenging. In many places, chemotherapy and radiation therapy are provided to slow the growth of the cancer but do not offer great hopes of cure. But a second surgery is complicated, mainly because the patient's anatomy is pretty messed up from the first surgery, making the subsequent surgery complex to plan and execute. Mayo was willing to take it on. So the band got back together for a do-over. I had appointments with all of the same physicians who had treated me earlier—Thor, Michael, Scott—and by the time I arrived they had already discussed my case at a tumor board.

A second thing that became clear this time was that I was better equipped to be more actively engaged in my care. For example, during Cancer 1.0 I had learned that a temporary ostomy wasn't fun, so I definitely wanted to avoid having a permanent one. Somehow I convinced myself that the second surgery might not involve removal of more of my colon. However, at a joint appointment with Thor and Scott I received the bad news that because the tumor was attached to the outside of my colon, I would need to have more of that organ removed. Thor, Scott, and both of their nurses sat quietly with me for a very long time while I processed my disappointment, waiting for me to ask questions but not making me move on until I was ready. Their silent witnessing was a remarkable gift.

I remember zeroing in on that issue: if I had to have more of my gut removed, I really didn't want an ostomy. I was balancing quality of life versus length of life. Scott heard me and made no promises, but I was clear in my mind—if I could avoid having an ostomy, that's what I wanted, even if it marginally increased my chances of another cancer recurrence.

I talked about my ostomy aversion with Ed and one or two very close friends who didn't like my decision and tried to talk me out of it. They wanted me to take the most aggressive pathway I could toward beating cancer. Those conversations helped me understand, viscerally, why people want to take control of their medical situation, and how, why, and when people with more advanced cancers may conclude that they are done fighting the disease.

My chemotherapy started in February 2021. It was a different formula this time, something called FOLFIRI, but the duration was the same—another eight rounds over sixteen weeks. Midway through chemotherapy, I had another PET scan and an MRI to determine whether the tumor was shrinking or growing and to get specific imaging requested by different members of the surgical team.

After chemo, I had radiation therapy in June and July 2021. For Cancer 2.0, I asked if I was a candidate for proton therapy, rather than photon therapy. A proton beam is more targeted and does less damage to adjacent areas of the body. Michael agreed, and I had fifteen rounds of therapy, a session every weekday for three weeks.

Receiving proton beam therapy was even more sci-fi than getting photon therapy. Four large, darkened treatment rooms in the proton beam facility are connected to a single shared giant cyclotron in the bowels of the building that produces a constant stream of protons. I was placed on a tall movable table, positioned precisely using X-rays, the machinery making *Star Wars*–appropriate sounds. While I'd been partially clothed during my previous cancer treatment, this time I was naked from the chest down except for a small towel over my loins. When it was my turn for the beam, I got zapped for a few seconds. During the thirty seconds that it took to reposition me for a second blast from another angle, the beam was switched to one of the adjacent treatment rooms—the cyclotron never rests. Then it came back to me for a second stream of billions of protons smashing into the tumor.

In early July, I began to meet the extended surgical team. In addition to Scott from colorectal surgery, the surgical team also included members from urology, vascular surgery, orthopedics, plastic surgery, and radiation oncology. Each described their roles and the risks to me.

On July 14, I had my last radiation treatment. That brought me to my lifetime limit for exposure to radiation therapy. Any more radiation treatments would put me at risk of developing leukemia or another form of cancer due to excess exposure to radiation.

I checked into the hospital for a preliminary vascular surgery to block the left internal iliac artery and vein to avoid excessive bleeding during surgery. That same day I checked directly into Mayo Methodist Hospital and began a colonoscopy prep. The next morning at 7:00, the medical transport team collected me and rolled me to the pre-surgical area. All my surgeons came by to visit as I got final prep for surgery. At 8:00 I was wheeled into the same operating room where I had been twenty-eight months earlier. A mask was placed over my mouth and nose, and I lost consciousness.

When I emerged from anesthesia after sixteen hours of surgery, I had the alarming, dreamy illusion that my arms and legs were being sutured into a large machine and I was being made part of some awful Borg. My eyes were still shut. I felt my abdomen with my hands. I knew that if there was a bag on the right, it was a temporary ostomy; if it was on the left, I would have an ostomy for the rest of my life. I couldn't find the bag, so I asked the nurses where it was. They said I didn't have one because Dr. Kelley had hand-sewn my large intestine back together. I was coherent enough to think, *Thank you, Scott.* But something was still wrong, because I couldn't feel or move my left leg or left hand. I kept trying to explain this to the nurses with the drunken incoherence of someone just emerging from anesthesia.

Eventually I was transported to a hospital room. I had two surgical drains protruding from my abdomen, an IV in my arm, a catheter, an oxygen tube in my nose, the familiar inflatable booties squeezing my legs, and a bed that inflated and deflated to keep me from getting bed sores. The surgical teams came to check on me and explain what had happened during surgery. The urologist explained that the tumor was located very close to the ureter connecting my left kidney to my bladder, and the ureter had been badly damaged from radiation. So they'd constructed a new ureter using tissue from my bladder and rebuilt my bladder.

Orthopedics had responsibility for managing surgery near certain nerves. With the anesthesia having mostly worn off, I finally was able to convey coherently that I couldn't move my left hand or leg. The orthopedic surgeons examined me to check the extent of paralysis in my left leg (I could move my foot just a little) and determine why my left hand could squeeze weakly but otherwise was numb and motionless. The conclusion was that nerves to my leg through my pelvis had been impaired by being moved and compressed during surgery, and then further damaged by radiation therapy delivered to the area of my tumor during the surgery itself. My hand was probably paralyzed because of the way I had been strapped to the table during my sixteen-hour surgery. Would I recover the use of my leg and arm? Everyone said they hoped so, but it was uncertain.

For the next two weeks I was visited daily by Dr. Kelley or a member of his team. I was really grateful for their visits, even when they occurred at 6:00 or 7:00 a.m., because my recovery was much more difficult than the first time. I developed a blood clot in my left arm, which swelled mightily, so I needed to have it tightly wrapped most of the time. And just like after my first surgery, I developed an ileus, when my intestines stopped moving food through them. This time I needed a nasogastric (NG) tube inserted to continually empty my stomach. (It's necessary but extremely unpleasant.) I couldn't eat or drink for twelve days. To be certain I didn't have blood clots in my leg or fluid in my abdomen, I was imaged repeatedly. A third drain was inserted into my abdomen to remove fluid. I was visited frequently by orthopedics and neurology, who checked every day for any reduction in paralysis. Physical therapists helped me stand and walk a few steps with the support of a leg brace—a brave undertaking on their part, as I am six foot five and towered over them unsteadily. Occupational therapy tried to help me regain motion in my hand.

Through all this I couldn't walk at all, and until I was taught how to stand on my good leg and pivot myself from bed to chair, I had to be moved from place to place with a ceiling crane and a harness. A shower was a ninety-minute odyssey managed only with the calm and kind support of medical assistants. To distract and amuse myself, I started to count how many people had seen me naked during this ordeal; I stopped counting when I got to twenty. Through all of this, the calmness, empathy, and professionalism of the nurses, phlebotomists, medical assistants, techs, physical therapists, occupational therapists, and physicians was truly amazing. I felt understood and supported. I was intensely grateful and thanked people constantly.

I was also very grateful for visitors—Ed came to see me on day three, and it was truly joyful to be distracted and to have a chance to talk about this book. Emily came to visit about every other day, driving 160 miles round-trip from St. Paul. Other visitors came as well, and everyone seemed able to ignore the tube up my nose, the IV in my arm, the catheter draining my bladder, and the surgical drains taking fluid from my belly.

Near the end of my two-week stay in the colorectal unit, I had a learning experience about advocating for oneself. The nasogastric tube into my stomach had been in place for a few days, but my intestines showed no sign of returning to normal function. Scott had told me that it was very difficult to predict when an ileus would occur and when it would end. He told me of one patient who spent a month in the hospital, going for long walks every day with his wife, waiting for his ileus to end. The nurse who had placed my NG tube was amazingly competent, but it was a bit of an ordeal, and I didn't want to do it a second time. For that reason, I didn't want the tube to come out until it was clear that my intestines had restarted.

On a Sunday morning, a colorectal surgery resident came to tell me it was time to take out the nasogastric tube. Residents have completed medical school and are doctors, but they are still early in their training and are rotating through various specialties learning different fields of medicine. This resident explained to me what a nasogastric tube was (I wanted to say, *Hello—the tube and I have become close friends, since it's been down my throat for about ten days*) and that it was time to take it out. I asked how they knew I didn't still need it. I expected an answer describing evidence that my ileus had ended, but instead the resident repeated in the same eighth-grade language that it was time to take it out. The resident was asking me to suspend judgment, ask no questions, and follow orders. But I was having none of it. I said I wanted evidence the ileus had ended before agreeing to have the tube come out. The resident again said only that the tube needed to come out. We repeated that cycle two or three times before I finally said, "OK, we've reached a deadlock here. I want evidence before I agree to have it taken out, and I will decide. I hear you say it's time for it to be removed, but I don't think you're hearing me." The resident seemed flustered and probably felt like a failure for not getting the result that Dr. Kelley, the supervising physician, had asked them to accomplish. I said I would be willing to talk more if the resident could answer my questions, but without answers I felt done discussing it. The tube stayed in place.

The next day, Monday, Dr. Kelley came by on rounds. "I heard you and my resident had a conversation about removing your NG tube."

"Yup."

He chuckled. "We'll take it out when you're ready," he said. "But here's what I think would show you don't need it anymore." We could test it by periodically stopping the tube and letting me drink some water, then measuring how much came out of the tube. It all made perfect sense to me. A few days later, I said I thought the tube could come out.

There's never anything wrong about speaking up for yourself and making sure your questions are answered. Sometimes it might not feel good, though. Even though this resident was about the age of my daughters and did not seem terribly experienced with the issue at hand or fully confident in patient communications, I still felt powerless as I lay in bed, barely able to manage my own body. But I felt I needed to advocate for myself and trust my ability to understand the logic and the data in the situation and express my own judgment about the conclusions.

Rehab

After two weeks, I was transferred to the inpatient rehabilitative medicine unit. The program was goal-oriented—intended to get me home and equip me for life as is, and perhaps to improve my function. Emblematic of the whole thing were morning rounds, where the entire team would come to each room. A facilitator would read out the goals for the day and what was needed to move me toward being ready for discharge. Everyone would chime in as appropriate.

The first few days were challenging. On day two, I developed a second ileus in the middle of the night. Images were taken, and the nurse on duty said I needed another nasogastric tube. I liked this nurse and felt he was very competent, but I asked whether he had placed a nasogastric tube recently (since this was a physical rehab unit, not a gastrointestinal unit). He told me he used to do them frequently in a previous healthcare institution but admitted that it had been a couple of years. He suggested I think about it while he went to reread the Mayo protocol to make sure he was doing it the Mayo way. I agreed to have it done. Partway through I had a somewhat painful sensation and felt I couldn't breathe. I was able to choke out "I think it's gone into my lung," and he promptly removed it and apologized. Recalling my earlier patient self-advocacy around nasogastric tubes, I said, "No offense, I think you're a great nurse, but could we possibly find someone from a GI floor who does this all the time?" To his credit, he did exactly what I asked for. A nurse arrived at about 3:30 a.m. from a GI unit elsewhere in the hospital and placed the tube with plenty of gagging and vomiting but without any additional drama.

When I went to my first physical therapy session in a big, sun-filled gym-like room with all kinds of specialty equipment, I wanted to heal but wasn't sure how I could. I arrived there in a surgical gown with three drains hanging from my belly and clipped to my hospital gown, an IV in my arm, a nasogastric tube taped to my face, and a catheter and bag strapped to the walker I was using. They put me into a leg brace and asked me to take twenty, then thirty, then fifty steps. *How can I do this?* I looked around the room and saw some of my fellow patients: people with severe trauma injuries, who'd had strokes, or were recovering from brain and spinal surgeries. All of us were just doing what we could, as hard as we could. Many people were in much worse shape than I was. I just put trust in the process and committed to bring my best to my own healing.

I ordered some running shorts from Amazon and had them delivered to my room, so I could do my work in workout clothes rather than a hospital gown. I went to two classes a day, just putting one foot in front of the other. In between I watched the oddly deserted summer Olympic Games in Tokyo, delayed one year because of the pandemic. Somehow I found it really reassuring to watch world-class athletes even though I was still a paralyzed, limp, catheterized mess.

For the next two weeks I had physical therapy and occupational therapy twice a day. After a few days one drain was removed, then another. Because of a small setback I had another drain placed just above my left buttock, which hurt. In physical therapy I learned to use a leg brace, how to use crutches and a wheelchair, and how to go up and down stairs. But my leg remained paralyzed. In occupational therapy they tried many things to wake up my hand—arm and hand exercises, electric stimulation, vibration. I remember the bizarre, almost nightmarish experience of staring at my hand, trying as hard as I could to get it to move, with nothing happening.

Near the end of my rehabilitation, I still had no muscle function in my left leg and hand. I was fitted for a custom leg brace made of white plastic extending from my butt to my foot—I looked like a half-dressed *Star Wars* stormtrooper—that locked my leg into a fully extended position. I wore a hand brace to keep my hand from just flopping around. But I now could walk up and down stairs. I could use crutches to go long distances. I could speed around in a wheelchair. We mocked up a little space in the bathroom the dimensions of my shower at home and rehearsed how I was going to get in and out without falling. I learned how to use a computer keyboard with one hand. All my drains, tubes, and catheters had been removed. I had begun to emerge as an independent human being after a month in the hospital being dependent on others for even the most basic functions.

On a sunny Saturday morning, August 13, I was discharged from the hospital. Hannah had flown in from Seattle, and she and Emily carried all my bags to the waiting car. The nurse who managed my discharge accepted a hug in appreciation for the care I had received. I had been looking for milestones and incentives to help keep me motivated. As the discharge date became more certain, my goal was to attend a big outdoor Irish fair with my daughters, an event we had loved visiting together before. On Sunday, my daughters and I drove to the fair and parked with my newly issued handicapped parking tag. They pushed me in a wheelchair as we watched Irish dancing, checked out the shops in the tents, and ate Irish food. We toasted to life together as we listened to an Irish punk band. Looking back, I can see that I was barely functional—in a wheelchair, wearing leg and hand braces, experiencing pain, and unable to do much because of my limited stamina. But on that sunny Sunday with my daughters, I finally celebrated being cancer-free, being alive and taking a few steps down the road to health. I could not work on my healing if I could not envision a life with joy. On that day I felt true joy being outside in the sunshine, feeling as though I had escaped from being devoured by cancer, able to imagine a joyful life even as I acknowledged that I might never walk normally again or regain function in my hand.

Continuing to Heal

Over the next nine months, I continued outpatient physical and occupational therapy at a great facility in Minneapolis. After three months, my left hand began to move a tiny bit, then more, and then with some strength. In mid-December, after therapists applied things like electrical stimulation, the leg muscles in the front of my left thigh, the quadriceps, slowly began to function again. By February I had enough leg muscle function that I graduated to a flexible leg brace and walking poles. More muscles in my leg returned to function. By March I could walk without a leg brace or walking poles. What an improvement from the fear that I might be permanently disabled!

At this writing, I still don't have any feeling in my left thumb or forefinger, but my hand works well enough. I have very limited feeling in my leg, though I see some signs of potential further recovery, and

I've learned how to walk miles in a day even though I have a limp. My digestive system doesn't always work right with a couple of feet of colon missing and lots of scar tissue. But I'm finding new ways to be increasingly active around my limitations.

On my one-year anniversary after surgery I received confirmation that I was cancer free. I had a colonoscopy, a CT scan of my chest and abdomen, and a blood test that detects residual tumor DNA in my bloodstream and can predict whether I might develop cancer again. All were clear. As we are finishing the writing of this book in winter 2024, I have now had seven regularly scheduled exams, and I remain cancer free.

Writing this chapter wasn't easy, and I imagine it might be uninteresting to some and hard to read for others. I'm not someone who usually shares these kinds of details. But I am sharing them here with the intent of benefiting people who are facing serious illness and helping the people who care for them. Serious illness can be terrifying, messy, and dehumanizing. I hope my story is an example of how it is possible to persevere, speak up for yourself, make decisions, and find wells of resilience.

The inescapable truth is that you can't decide whether you are going to have a serious illness. You can live a healthy life, but that doesn't prevent you from getting sick. Ed is a world-class athlete who lives a very healthy life, but he still faced two major health crises, as you'll see in the next chapter. I was a thirty-year vegetarian with no lifestyle or genetic risks for rectal cancer, and I got it twice.

When everything else seems out of control, the only thing you can control is how you respond to your situation. Later in the book we are going to provide more specifics about how we think this is possible, even under the most frightening and adverse conditions.

Three

Double Trouble

When illness and career
collided for Ed Marx

U p until 2018 at age fifty-two, I was the picture of perfect health. In fact, my physician would often say how boring I was as a patient. I took no medications and had no illnesses. Other than a couple of sport-specific injuries along the way, I rarely visited a hospital outside of routine exams. I always made exercise, eating well, and trying to live a balanced life a priority. I had climbed several of the world's tallest peaks, completed in over a hundred triathlons, including several Ironman contests, and led one of the top adventure race teams in the country, named after the health system most of the team served with, Texas Health. I rarely sat still.

Despite my good health and prognosis, over the next two years I faced death twice, with the two leading killers of men: heart attack and cancer. I have now learned that life and health are fragile and fickle. Even if a clinician says everything you want to hear in terms of your health, you are still responsible and must be ready to deal with challenges that can arise.

The Widowmaker

My wife, Simran, is a nurse through and through, and she's always loved how active I am. She also has always insisted that I get routine and sophisticated exams to ensure that my body can keep up with all my athletic pursuits. In March 2018, I had an all-day intensive "executive physical," one of the perks of being a Cleveland Clinic executive. I spent the day in a wellness setting, where I had ten to fifteen clinical appointments back to back, complete with lab work and imaging studies. Given my affinity for sports, clinicians took specific measures of my heart. I underwent numerous tests ranging from simple blood work to rigorous stress tests, where they forced me to run to exhaustion as they looked for any signs of abnormalities. At the end of it all, there was a review of my results and a debriefing with the lead clinician. At age fifty-two, I was given a clean bill of health and told I was in the top 1 percent of men in my age group when it came to all the markers clinicians look for when evaluating health, wellness, and risks. I left feeling confident about my health and unworried when it came to my extreme-sports lifestyle. Of course, that was exactly what I'd wanted to hear, so I left no room in my mind for the possibility that something could go wrong.

One month after my executive physical, I was running the last two miles of the Team USA Duathlon National Championships in Greenville, South Carolina. Duathlon is a multisport event where you run, cycle, and then run a second time. Team USA is the governing body for the Olympic sport of triathlon; they organize official race events where participants of all ages can compete against the country's best athletes. Athletes who finish at the top of their age group qualify for Team USA and represent their country at annual world championships.

The overall top finishers are named to the Olympic team. I was in a position to make Team USA for the fifth straight year when I suddenly felt a tightness in my chest.

I told myself it could not be a heart attack. I was still running about a 6:30 mile, and I had no other symptoms. Plus I'd just had my executive physical and had been told that I was in top condition. At the same time, I was smart enough to know that something was happening. As I continued to run, I began to self-triage. I reasoned that if I stopped, by the time medical help got to me, too much precious time might be lost, and I knew that every minute of delay meant that heart muscle could be damaged or lost. Part of me was in denial: how bad could it be if I was still able to run? But another part of me knew. The debate went on in my head as I powered to the end of the race.

The ambulance and medical personnel were all at the medical tent next to the finish line. There, the same digital health tools I promoted as part of my work at Cleveland Clinic were the tools that diagnosed me and saved my life. I checked myself in and we connected a credit card–sized EKG (measuring the electrical activity of my heart) to my iPhone and transferred the results to the local designated Team USA hospital. They responded: "Bring him in, stat! He is having a massive heart attack." My left anterior descending (LAD) artery was completely blocked. A blockage there is called a widowmaker because 90 percent of the time it causes instant death.

At the hospital I met the doctor and his team. Thankfully, they were at the hospital early that Saturday morning because they had already had an emergency case before me. The doctor was very reassuring and explained the entire procedure in detail. I watched on the big screen as the interventional cardiologist snaked a tiny balloon catheter through my artery, opened up the blocked blood vessel, and installed a stent. My heart reawakened and began to dance as blood poured in unobstructed. The pressure on my chest lifted.

I was bewildered by what had just happened. I thought the tests and my lifestyle had proved how healthy my heart was. But I later learned that despite my having above-average test results and the benefits of exercise, acute physical stress (that is, intense exercise) or emotional stress can cause a heart attack. How? One theory put forward in the *Journal of the American Medical Association* (*JAMA*) is that acute exertion may cause plaque in a coronary artery to rupture. My clinicians think that while I was running, what little arterial plaque I did have was dislodged, and that caused a chain reaction of events that quickly blocked my left anterior descending artery, leading to the heart attack. While very unusual in otherwise healthy individuals, it does sometimes happen—and it sure happened to me.

Planning to Race Again

In the recovery room after the procedure, I asked my wife if I'd made Team USA. Simran shook her head, in disbelief that I would even ask such a question. But she told me that because I'd finished, I remained in the top ten and qualified for the world championships ninety days later in Odense, Denmark.

Out loud I said: "Not only am I alive, but I made the team again. Now, can I recover in time to race?" I was kind of trying to be funny, but deep down I really wanted to know.

Back at Cleveland Clinic, the clinicians laughed at the thought that I might recover from a LAD heart attack in time to race in Denmark.

They told me to be happy if I could walk the distance, never mind run and bike it. But I resolved to wear the red, white, and blue racing outfit and to continue to represent our country, my streak uninterrupted.

I pushed them. I insisted on leveraging new technologies. They agreed to monitor all my digital data and change treatments as needed. Indeed, the lead cardiologist was adjusting my medication regimen on a near-daily basis for the first several weeks.

Had I not insisted that the clinicians adopt the latest tools, my recovery would have been normal, but truly suboptimal. Unacceptable, really. Given my pre-widowmaker activity levels, being restricted for a long period of time for recovery would have impacted my mental state more than my physical state. I was scared clinicians would insist on minimal activity or put me on traditional medicine protocols that only looked to make adjustments every few weeks. I wanted changes to be made every few days! I got them because I insisted. This is what's known as "shared decision-making," a concept we will hit on a few times later in this book. Patients and their families should be involved in all medical decisions. And you can push for what you want. In fact, you should—respectfully, kindly, but clearly.

Simran ensured I took no shortcuts or otherwise deviated from my customized plan. As my cardiovascular function continued to improve, the clinicians allowed me to progress from walking to brisk walking to jogging and ultimately running.

Ninety days after my heart attack, I raced for Team USA at the world championships. As I neared the finish line, I heard our Team USA coach yell my name. He stretched his hand into the running lane and gave me an American flag. I crossed the finish line with that mighty red, white, and blue hoisted high in the air, and I cried hard as I did.

So did my clinical team when I recounted the story to them. If I had not taken charge of my recovery, my association with Team USA would have been nothing more than a memory of past glory. Nothing could be further from what's happened: I have qualified and raced for Team USA every year since.

While the location for the World Championships changes each year, the US national championships are normally held two years in a row in the same place. It was eerie returning to Greensboro in 2019 to race on the same course where I'd had that widowmaker. It turned out to be rather cathartic. I was a little scared at first, but here is what made the situation extra special. Prior to the race, I walked into the medical tent. Sure enough, there were the same doctor and nurses who'd taken care of me one year prior. They had not forgotten me, nor I them. We had a tearful reunion. While I had sent cards and memorabilia to all involved in my care the year prior, I hadn't yet been able to say thank you in person. That day I did. Actually I don't think I got past my introduction before we all started hugging and crying. Words were unnecessary. Thankfully, the race went well, and I had no reason to return to their tent.

After this experience, Simran and I figured we could handle anything life might throw at us. Little did we expect that the following year I would have to battle another life-threatening health condition and contend with a whole new patient experience.

Cancer

It was 6:35 a.m. when I walked into Cleveland Clinic's corporate offices on June 10, 2019. In the lobby was an expressionless Dr. Eric Klein, chair of the Gluckman Urology and Kidney Institute. We both knew why he was there. Two days prior, we'd met in his office to discuss the results of my prostate-specific antigen (PSA) test. That test suggested an extremely high probability of prostate cancer. The next day I'd undergone an invasive biopsy to determine if I had cancer or not. Clearly the results were in.

Without saying a word, I motioned to him to follow me into my office. I sat down and took a deep breath before making eye contact.

"Ed, it's not the news I was hoping to give you," Dr. Klein said. "You have Gleason level 7 prostate cancer." He spent the next few minutes elaborating on the diagnosis and available treatment options, none of them good. I thanked him, and awkwardly we gathered our belongings and walked together down the hall to the 7:00 a.m. Thursday senior management meeting. At that point I had no idea what "Gleason level" meant, and I think I only retained a fraction of what he'd just shared. All I recall is "You have cancer." After the meeting was called to order, I quietly stepped out and called Simran. She cried. Simran and I met Dr. Klein the following Monday to finalize treatment decisions.

My mother died of ovarian cancer in 2004. A Holocaust survivor and mother of seven, she put up one hell of a fight. It was terribly ugly. By the time she traded her earthly rags for robes of righteousness, we were thankful. My father, the concentration camp escapee, is still kicking, two decades' worth of bone and skin cancer behind him. Assisting in their journeys had been rewarding, enlightening, and downright frightening for me. I *knew* what lay ahead.

Unlike my heart attack, which was a complete surprise, I'd had an inkling that this day of cancer reckoning was coming. My PSA score started going up in 2013, after I substantially increased the time I spent cycling. I was doing more than a hundred miles per week. The sitting position of a man on a bike seat puts an extraordinary amount of pressure on the prostate. Since there were no other symptoms, my physicians attributed the PSA increase to my cycling miles but decided to monitor for changes carefully. Each year at my annual physical we reviewed the PSA levels, and they continued to climb higher with each test. In 2017, my doctors recommended testing every six months, which we did, and still the levels continued to climb, but no further actions were recommended. To be honest, I just listened and followed the clinicians' judgment, never questioning it despite what, looking back, seem to have been obvious danger signs. Had I taken my own health more seriously when the warning signs first emerged in 2013, I would have discovered the cancer earlier, allowing for less-invasive treatment options. My blissful ignorance and my allowing the clinicians' assessment to be the absolute last word could have killed me.

My wife, Simran, would have no more of it, though. In 2018 she teamed up with my cardiologist during a follow up appointment after my widowmaker and they arranged for me to have an appointment with the urology institute chair. Dr. Klein's team had recently developed a new test to better predict the likelihood of prostate cancer. The morning after I took the test, Dr. Klein shared the result, which suggested that I had a 50 percent likelihood of cancer. He asked me to come in for the biopsy. At noon that day, I was in his exam room, backside exposed. Now that it appeared I really did have cancer, I wasted no time.

While the self-pity was still fresh, I reflected on the irony that my wife and I lived clean lives. Simran was winning fitness contests, and I was climbing mountains and running the world's toughest endurance races. I was a member of Team USA Triathlon. What else would it have taken, I wondered, to keep me from this fate?

That was when it became clear to me: cancer does not discriminate. It pays no attention to timing, either. I had recently had a heart attack—and now I had to deal with *cancer*? Why me?

Yep. I had to accept it, move on from the pity, and fight. Build resilience. But I discovered that as good a mantra as that was, I couldn't do it alone. And I was blessed that I didn't have to.

Simran and I called our children, as well as some of our closest family members. We shared the news with our best friends directly. I told my work team, whom I affectionately call my brothers and sisters, via email. I called my direct reports. There were lots of hugs. There were also lots of tears—but only from others. At that time, I had yet to shed a single tear.

Simran and I met with Dr. Klein to review options. My wife and I soon became experts in prostate health. We studied prostate cancer treatment options and reviewed outcomes so that, in conjunction with our clinical team, we could make the best possible decisions. These were the hallmarks of Cleveland Clinic: empathetic care and shared decision-making.

We concluded that the best long-term treatment for us was radical prostatectomy, the removal of the prostate. After gathering second opinions and research on open versus closed surgical techniques, we decided to stick with Dr. Klein. While he only used the traditional open approach, he is one of the world's best surgeons and a colleague and friend.

We decided not to rush the surgery date. That way, we could time the surgery to accommodate Simran's clinical rotation, and I could wrap up some strategic initiatives at work. In addition, we could attend the biannual Marx family reunion over the July 4 holiday. Surgery would follow shortly thereafter, giving me the rest of the summer to recover.

With the surgery date scheduled, life moved very fast. I did a lot of thinking in the days leading up to my surgery. I remembered a promise I had made to myself upon my mother's death, thirteen years prior. I'd vowed to live a life with no regrets. I would try new adventures that might kill me, learn how to dance, and pursue a life of faith and passion. More than once since then, I had failed to live up to my promise to myself—and others. Broken relationships, hurt feelings, kindnesses overlooked: there was plenty for me to beat myself up over. I took account of all my wrongdoings and reached out to make amends. Most people responded favorably, for which I was grateful.

I focused on making sure my team at work would continue to move forward boldly without me. They were strong and ready. It made me proud to see how ready they were.

Our best friends hosted a night of prayer and partying with some of our close friends. IT caregivers (everyone who works at Cleveland Clinic is called a caregiver instead of an employee) sent me hundreds of well-wishes on paper cutouts, which I hung in my office. I had a chance to catch up with my five children. The family reunion was the perfect occasion to hug some of the dearest people in my life. The outpouring of love from friends, family, and work colleagues was overwhelming. Simran and I were so thankful to be part of this village, which was there to hold us and love us and help carry the burdens.

The diagnosis of cancer brought me clarity and forced me to face my own mortality. My confidence in a complete recovery increased because I knew friends around the world were interceding on my behalf with positive thoughts and prayers. The ongoing love and support from fellow

Cleveland Clinic caregivers was palpable. Most importantly, Simran was amazing in her unwavering support and willingness to rearrange her life in order to nurse me back to health.

Over the weeks before my surgery, I examined myself the best I knew how. My character, my spirit, my actions—all of it. After introspection, analysis, research, and philosophical discussions, I thought I had found four verbs that define *me*, what I do and why I do it: *shape, study, share,* and *serve*. *Shape* has dual meanings. I am called to help shape people in their self-development and careers. It also means to take care of myself, emotionally, physically, and spiritually. *Study* is to always be in a learning mode. *Share* is to actively share what I learn with others so that they might grow also. Finally, *serve* is a reminder that I exist to serve others. I serve my family, my community, and my place of work.

After the surgery, there were lots of people asking questions and expressing genuine concern. I told them I was fine. It might have been denial, or my Germanic heritage may have made me go for a little stoic bravado in my darkest hour. But I wanted to believe it was confidence. I felt no regrets and no uncertainty. The surgery had gone well, thanks to Dr. Klein and his team, number one in the world.

While recovering, I posted memories and pictures daily on my Facebook feed. I had previously posted photos of the many high mountains I had climbed, and now I began to draw parallels between the perils and challenge of climbing and my cancer. I saw my battle with cancer as one more mountain, my Everest. Surgery was my base camp, where I could nourish myself, formulate a plan, and wait for the weather to clear. Then I would climb to the summit for healing. In other words, I was not done yet. Surgery was just a plateau of sorts. There were still challenges ahead.

In the days after the surgery, Simran and I continued to pray morning and night for a clean pathology report. Even while I was getting my catheter out, I could think of nothing but the one word that I wanted to hear. While we were waiting, I had some minor setbacks in my recovery. After the drains were pulled, I had recurring edema, and the drains had to be surgically reimplanted. They were a nuisance to clean and maintain. Only patients and their families know the rigors of surgical recovery, especially with open surgeries, where extensive cuts have been made into the body. There's the physical therapy, the maintenance of drains, the multitude of follow-up appointments, the difficulties involved in just bathing and taking care of yourself. It requires a village.

Cured

Simran and I were sitting on our living room couch on July 12, 2019, having just finished lunch, when I received an alert that a test result was available in my online patient portal. Simultaneously, Dr. Klein phoned. "Great news on your path," he said. "Cancer confined, cured. Congrats!"

That was it—the word I had been waiting to hear. *Cured.*

I stood up and wailed in the arms of my lover, my bestie, my cancer caretaker. My gratitude, expressed in tears and convulsive sobs, conveyed unspeakable joy. Cradled in the earthly bosom of God, I felt peace at last. Hearing Simran's shouts, our teenage daughter, Shalani, came to check on her parents. She joined our clutch. As we let go to breathe, Shalani wiped tears from my eyes. It was a moment I will not forget. I finally cried.

Over the next few weeks, my heart and mind returned to friends who had been stricken with cancer over the past few years. There were so many of them. I thought it fortunate that I could be there for them because I realized how much it meant to me that others had been there in my time of my need.

The annual Cleveland Clinic VeloSano "Bike to Cure" cancer cycling fundraiser was around the corner. Given my post-surgery condition, I would be unable to ride with my Cleveland Clinic IT cycling squad. We had ridden together the year prior and raised a lot of money to help cure cancer, but we'd had even higher hopes for this year. I was sad thinking that I'd have to miss that. But then they sent me an email:

> Ed, many of us have been following your cancer journey. As outsiders to this ordeal, your candor and level of detail have been fascinating to follow. No one can be more grateful/thankful than you are for your cancer-free diagnosis. But we are all thankful the mountain of good intentions/wishes has paid off and you are on the road to recovery. For this year's VeloSano, the mighty VeloSano IT Team has agreed to wear a blue ribbon on our jerseys to honor you and your warrior battle to beat Prostate Cancer. The color blue symbolizes prostate cancer. We may not have been with you and your family on your cancer journey, but you and your cancer-fighting spirit will be on the 400+ miles the IT Team will pedal for cancer research this weekend. #ridetocure #marxstrong.

It was kindness, pure and simple. Kindness that made me cry and fueled my hope.

There were many more challenges to follow. The first two were my bladder and erectile dysfunction. I was grateful that my bladder function had returned right after the nurse removed my catheter. It had been humbling putting men's diapers in our Target shopping cart, and I was thankful I never needed them; at the same time, my heart went out to those not as fortunate. Overcoming erectile dysfunction took a while longer, but Dr. Klein said I had the quickest recovery he'd ever seen.

My cancer journey attuned me to the feeling of fear, of not knowing what was around the corner and of no longer being in control. I felt a loss of dignity. I knew the desire to eliminate pain. At the same time, I learned the joy of a friendly face coming to console me and how to appreciate the loving feelings that came from receiving all kinds of flowers. I appreciated the work the clinicians did and their dedication to my case.

Cancer-free, I would continue to serve a world-class organization, alongside the best clinicians, educators, and researchers. *That* propelled me onward, along with all the love that I was feeling.

At my five-week postoperative visit, Dr. Klein shared more good news: my PSA level was zero. I was indeed cured.

A Healthcare Executive's Lessons Learned

Make no mistake—throughout my heart attack and recovery process and my battle with cancer, I was paying attention to how my experience as a patient related to my role as a healthcare executive. While I had a superb theoretical understanding of all the things that patients experience, there was no comparison to actually being a patient. Especially a patient with serious health problems. While I never leveraged my organizational position during my treatment, I was wise enough to understand that as challenging as my journeys were, I had a clear advantage over other patients. I had an insider's knowledge of how healthcare worked in all of its glorious dysfunction, and that softened the hard edges. I understood the why behind various clinical decisions and processes. I knew that some decisions were outside the hospital's control and based on insurance rules and government regulations. I knew where and when to push and advocate for myself. Even so, healthcare's gaps in providing a quality patient and family experience were fully exposed.

After my prostate surgery, when I was transferred from the operating room to recovery, my wife was appropriately notified and was debriefed by our surgeon. The recovery room nurse, however, failed to inform Simran of my status and never allowed her to visit once I was awake. I recall asking the nurse if I could see my wife, and she said she was tracking her down. The entire time I lay in recovery I was anxious to see Simran and she was anxious to see me. There was a complete breakdown in process and communication with the recovery room team and my wife.

It got worse. I was moved from the recovery room to my hospital bed in a different part of the hospital. The recovery room team failed to tell Simran of my move. When she kept asking to see me, one of the nurses, realizing the communications breakdown, apologized and tried to help Simran find where I had been resettled. Nobody seemed to have any idea. We were now two-plus hours post-surgery, and I still had not seen my wife. We were finally reunited around the three-hour mark, but only after Simran had lodged numerous complaints and asked to speak to directors and vice presidents.

Despite having world-class care in an organization known for its high-quality patient experience, we were having a nightmare at our most vulnerable time. The fact that I, not just a healthcare executive but an executive in the organization that was treating me, had such a terrible experience made me wonder what it is like for the average patient. If this can happen to me, it can happen to any other patient.

In hindsight, I am thankful for that dose of reality. It was one reason I was motivated to write this book and to share with you my hard-won insights into what patients need to know and do to make sure they receive optimal medical and patient care. My two journeys through the healthcare system have taught me that, as a patient, you have to cultivate the attitude and belief that *you* are in charge and not be afraid to challenge those in authority. You must be proactive in all aspects of your care and experience.

My post-heart-attack recovery is a good example of how that approach bestows enormous benefits. Had I followed the traditional path that the medical team was recommending, my care would have been suboptimal. Instead, I took charge and asked the clinicians to treat me differently and to leverage the latest technology available. They did. I healed more quickly, and my lifestyle greatly improved.

Before I had to become a patient, I already wielded a fair amount of influence on our organization's attitude about maximizing the patient experience, but afterward, I was on a mission. I felt a sense of urgency and moral obligation to take more action and push harder than ever to improve on what was already a pretty decent patient-centric environment at Cleveland Clinic. I knew we could do more.

Another, equally important lesson from my two healthcare crises is that family and friends—as well as acquaintances and work colleagues—can be an enormous help in facing a diagnosis, handling a treatment process, and maximizing recovery. I am certain my outcomes would not have been as positive if I hadn't had this village around me to provide physical and emotional support. Having one or more close friends and family members who comfort you, talk with your doctors, let you express your worries, and help you understand what is happening to you brings needed peace and comfort. That's why I believe that one of the toughest tasks some people face as patients is being able to reach out and let those who care about them know they need their help and support. Being tough and strong—a good self-advocate—doesn't mean you can't let others know you need help.

Four

Your Discussions with You

All health journeys begin with you. Receiving a significant health diagnosis can be upsetting, shocking, life-changing. And after being diagnosed comes a time to confront real but unpleasant truths, to prepare yourself for the journey, to respond to difficulties and fears, and to relate to the people around you.

Your diagnosis may not be the result of any choices you made. You certainly would not choose to receive such a significant diagnosis. All you can choose is how to respond to this development in your life. Now is the time to have a discussion with yourself and decide what you want to do.

Some people try to control their health journeys; some feel better "trusting the process." Some people adopt realistic stoicism; some choose denial. In our journeys, we adopted a mix of styles. Sometimes we wanted very much to be in control; at other times we placed our trust in experts and in our family and friends to decide what should come next.

No matter what, you can't escape your role in your healing and wellness. You must participate in your journey. Regardless of how you want to engage in—or disengage from—your own health story, and regardless of the eventual outcome of the journey, we believe four things are essential for a positive healthcare experience:

- You need to know that the journey begins with you.
- You need to build resilience.
- You need to gain awareness.
- You need to put the pieces together.

Know That the Journey Begins with You

Whether you take an active role in managing your journey or take a more passive role in responding to events as they arise, self-acknowledgment is essential. Everything else—how you engage with your care team, how you build your community, and who you are at this moment—will depend on how you want to identify with your journey.

For the two of us, at least, it took some time to fully absorb that our diagnoses were real, to acknowledge that they were happening to us and not someone else, and to realize that we had to participate fully and actively in decisions about our care. Only when you have really owned up to your condition will you be in a good place to communicate with your care team and discern who is in your village and how to engage with them. But you come first. Just you.

Ed's solo journey: When I heard the words "You have cancer," my first thought was to dutifully comply with everything my clinician told me. After all, he is the expert. And I was scared. I knew if I followed his recommendations, the odds would be in my favor. But it wasn't that easy. My clinician presented me with many treatment choices and ultimately, I had to decide.

I wanted the clinician to tell me what to do. He wouldn't. He believed that he should give me good counsel and answer all my questions.

I also knew that while Simran was helpful, I could not make her bear the responsibility of making my treatment decision. I would need to own that decision and then live with it.

I finally accepted the fact that I alone needed to make the decision about treatment. My cancer journey would begin with me. And end with me. I did not want to become an expert in prostate cancer, but I had no other viable option. Rather than allow this new reality to discourage me, I decided to let the situation empower me to take charge and battle and win. That resolve gave me some seeds of hope and optimism.

Cris's solo journey: All my life I was healthy, and then I was pushed into the deep end of the pool—I had stage 3 rectal cancer. At first I treated it as "a problem to be solved," not "my problem." For me, the change came when a nurse described details about installation of a port for chemotherapy. I finally had to accept the reality that I was getting cancer treatment. They were going to do something to me.

When you accept that this—whatever health challenge it is—is happening to you and you have to confront it and shape your response to it, then you are ready to go on to the next step: resilience.

Build Resilience

Resilience is the ability to absorb hard news, endure difficult experiences, face fears, and respond with capacity and strength. A tough situation can become a good, manageable, or bad experience—depending on whether you can find, foster, and act with resilience or not.

Resilience has been well studied, and research suggests not just that many people have deep wells of resilience to tap but also that almost anyone can learn how to be more resilient.

We believe resilience is a key predictor of your experience as a patient. The more resilient you are, the greater the opportunity for a positive experience.

Research at Mayo Clinic recommends six ways that someone can become more resilient:

- **Get connected.** Building strong, positive relationships with loved ones and friends can provide you with needed support, guidance, and acceptance in good and bad times. Establish other important connections by volunteering or joining a faith or spiritual community.
- **Make every day meaningful.** Do something that gives you a sense of accomplishment and purpose every day. Set clear, achievable goals to help you look toward the future with meaning.
- **Learn from experience.** Think of how you've coped with hardships in the past. Consider the skills and strategies that helped you through difficult times. You might even write about past experiences in a journal to help you identify positive and negative behavior patterns and guide your future behavior.
- **Remain hopeful.** You can't change the past, but you can always look toward the future. Accepting and even anticipating change makes it easier to adapt and view new challenges with less anxiety.

- **Take care of yourself.** Tend to your own needs and feelings. Participate in activities and hobbies you enjoy. Include physical activity in your daily routine. Get plenty of sleep and create consistent bedtime rituals. Eat a healthy diet. Practice stress management and relaxation techniques, such as yoga, meditation, guided imagery, deep breathing, or prayer.
- **Be proactive.** Don't ignore your problems. Instead, figure out what needs to be done, make a plan, and take action. Although it can take time to recover from a major setback, traumatic event, or loss, know that your situation can improve if you work at it.

Ed's resilience journey: After my heart attack, as I lay flat on my back staring at the ceiling of the ambulance whisking me away from the race to the designated athletes' hospital, everything seemed as surreal as surreal can get. The ever-present siren assaulted my senses as we snaked through the streets on our way to the waiting trauma team. As my shock at what had happened faded, I was left with nothing but reality.

First, I was happy to be alive and stabilized. Second, I made a deal with my Maker and promised to become a better, more loving person. Third, I reckoned I had two choices for survival. One: embrace the situation and fight like hell. Or two: let things unfold however they would. I decided to embrace the situation and fight. Given my healthcare background, I knew the odds were slim that I would survive and be strong enough to race again, but this is what I resolved to do.

For me resilience became a choice. It is not a magical word or something you are born with. I discovered you can develop resilience.

My parents are Holocaust survivors, my dad a concentration camp escapee. I learned resilience as I saw them make a great life out of the fires of Auschwitz. I learned resilience participating in the ravages of my mom's ovarian cancer battle, which she ultimately lost. I learned resilience as a youngster moving from Bavaria to the United States at age ten. I absolutely did not fit in. I was picked on and bullied, and so I resolved to outsmart and outmaneuver my attackers. I did. I went on to shine in sports and create my own safe community of friends. Even in my army and early civilian careers it was the same. I never really fit the mold, but I leveraged resilience so that my naysayers could not hold me back. I sought to outperform and outhustle them. I ultimately outflanked and outranked them. That built my resilience. I never gave up, accepting everything as a challenge and believing I had some control in the process and outcome.

Riding in that ambulance, I thought of all the people who had told me I would never amount to much. Their names and faces were clear despite the years that had passed. Certain teachers. Certain coaches. Bullies. Some of my peers. I had beaten them when I was younger. I would beat this.

By the time the ambulance backed up to the emergency department entrance, I was already in the hospital in my spirit and mind. I told myself, "I will fight this, and not just survive but thrive. I will race in the world championships in ninety days. I will come back stronger and faster. I will kick the crap out of this widowmaker."

Cris's resilience journey: *My lowest point was after the sixteen-hour surgery for my second cancer. I emerged pretty messed up. All I* *could take on at first was that if I was going to heal, I needed to make it happen, and the only guy for that job was my best self. I needed to find him.*

My best self is inspired by my family. My children-of-immigrants grandparents were proper, well mannered, and sometimes formal, but always gentle, warm, and loving people. Everything in my upbringing emphasized love, duty to each other, kindness, respect, decency, charity, and faith.

In my worst moment the best person I could imagine being was someone who would make my grandparents proud. So to the nurses and doctors caring for me, I responded with all the kindness, appreciation, and gratitude I could muster. I thanked everyone, asked for things politely, apologized to overworked nurses, and asked them how they were feeling that day. I liked these people authentically and remain deeply grateful, but the secret truth is that I did this as much for me as for them. My efforts to act with kindness and gratitude came from a desire to be more than the broken, smelly, swollen, unmoving mess that I was. By acting as my best self—as a good person that the people who raised me would be proud of—I felt more human, more alive, and more sure that someday I wouldn't be in that bed, that I would shed all the tubes, and that I would be able to walk again. If I had retreated into a pity party of victimhood—and believe me, some days I wanted to—I would not have been able to gain the strength I needed to achieve what I wanted.

Many of the six components of resilience listed earlier are interwoven into both of our stories. You have more resilience than you might think—if you approach it with intention. You may find it very easy to cultivate resilience, or you may have to look at the six attributes repeatedly and make a plan to incorporate them from day to day. You might be able to find your own wells of resilience, or you may need a trusted person to help you get there. There is no right or wrong way to cultivate and maintain resilience—but we do know it is essential.

Action-oriented people might resonate with the active aspects of resilience: get connected, take care of yourself, be proactive. But people who like to be in control may find some parts of resilience-building, like making every day meaningful and being hopeful, to be less actionable and perhaps elusive or even a little soft or weak.

Those who take a more passive role in responding to their healthcare journeys may be open to the more introspective parts of resilience but find it harder to take the action needed to build resilience.

Whether you take an active or passive stance, your opportunities for a better patient experience and outcome are directly correlated with how resilient you are and can become. Resilience helps you understand and respond effectively to your situation—to gain awareness.

Gain Awareness

We believe you should attempt to increase awareness about yourself and gain awareness about your diagnosis, treatment options, family situation, and financial considerations. You should build awareness about your care team and your community. The more aware you become, the more potential there is for continued and increased resilience—and that will give you reserves to call on if the pressures of your journey through illness toward wellness intensify.

Ed's awareness journey: After I resolved that my cancer journey started and ended with me, I realized I needed to arm myself with as much information as I could. To make the best decisions about my care, I needed to understand the implications of my cancer and the pros and cons of each choice I would face. I came up with the following checklist. Yours may be more or less expansive.

1. *Gather and consume all the resources given to you by your clinicians.*

2. *Conduct research on all available options. You can do the majority of this via the internet. Use only credible resources backed by peer-reviewed research.*

3. *Join support groups for your specific ailment and investigate their resources.*

4. *Talk to many patients like you, especially those who have completed their treatment. Look online and for in-person opportunities to interact.*

5. *Get a second opinion. I trusted my clinician implicitly but still sought a second opinion to discover if there was more to learn.*

6. *Examine holistic options as well. Sometimes a significant change in diet and/or exercise can have a material impact.*

7. *Remain humble and extend grace to everyone you meet and to those who help you.*

Once you have conducted your initial round of research into treatment options, write out your choices. List pros and cons for each. Share your research with friends and family. Gather their *additional thoughts and ideas. Then share your research and conclusions with your clinical care team. See what validation you might receive or what they think you got wrong.*

The goal is to have absolute confidence when you make your treatment decisions. This confidence fuels resilience. Gathering feedback and support from your village (friends, family) and care providers is essential for the best experience you can have.

Cris's awareness journey: When my primary care physician said, "I'm sorry, you have colorectal cancer," I immediately went into situation-awareness mode, like the CIO I am. I asked questions, decided on next steps, and stayed calm. It felt like a safe and natural way to respond to a very frightening situation.

In the two weeks after my first diagnosis, I reached out to medical colleagues for advice and insights. I found that the answers and insights began to repeat and layer. A few things worked for me:

1. *Gather whatever information you can. Some people might take in information in a completely brainy, analytical, cognitive way. Some people might accept it in an "emotional truth" kind of way. Regardless, don't be oblivious. Try to avoid slipping into major denial (a little denial is sometimes unavoidable and maybe even healthy). Pay attention. Build your treatment journey into the narrative of your entire life.*

2. *Decide what you want, as best you can. The experience I'd garnered as a CIO responding to crisis said, "Find a set of simple rules or heuristics, and follow them until the facts*

*change and the rules change." So my starting rules for cancer
were:*

- *Give me the most potent treatment available to kill
  cancer cells. I will endure side effects as long as I can in
  order to give me a chance at life.*

- *Minimize permanent impairment. Rectal cancer has some
  potentially very negative ramifications, like a permanent
  ostomy bag for managing body waste and disruption to
  bowel, bladder, and sexual function. I didn't ask my
  doctors to keep me from the unavoidable, but I ranked
  the avoidable—for example, I really didn't want a
  permanent ostomy, and I was willing to take some risks of
  cancer recurrence to avoid it.*

Put the Pieces Together

We believe these three attributes—acknowledging that this is your
journey, building resilience, and gaining awareness—are foundational
to a meaningful health journey. We also believe that they are mutually
supporting. Acknowledging that this journey begins with you allows
you to take the steps that will make you more resilient. Being more
resilient gives you strengths and skills to better place yourself in your
own journey. Being aware helps you take more personalized ownership
of your journey, and so on.

While you might want to hand over this often-burdensome journey
to someone else—a loved one, a clinician, or an organization such as a
hospital—it is yours. But you don't have to be alone. Relying on others
as partners can be a key to healing. Still, when all is said and done, it is
you who owns this journey.

The Long Road to Appropriate Care Starts with You

Ginger, seventy-one, has contended with multiple health issues, including chronic kidney disease, multiple myeloma, dialysis, and lupus. She has had quite a journey. She repeatedly encountered doctors who dismissed her symptoms as emotionally fueled instead of physical in nature. But her village helped her find the care she needed—and deserved.

Lupus was the first health issue. It took a long time to get diagnosed, but I was finally given an explanation for how I was feeling in 1988. I had to advocate pretty strongly for myself back then because they didn't even have a protocol for treating the disease. Even the doctor would say, "But you don't look sick."

Then I developed chronic kidney disease—and because I didn't like my kidney doctor I changed to another office, out of my healthcare plan. That nephrologist said, "Something is going on—how come nobody has followed through?"

She sent me to a hematologist-oncologist, and that was when I was diagnosed with monoclonal gammopathy of undetermined significance (MGUS), a blood disorder that affects plasma cells in your bone marrow. After repeated regular checkups to keep tabs on that, it progressed to smoldering myeloma.

I was already part of Mayo Connect, their forum for patients to support and inform each other, so I asked the group for recommendations for a top-notch doctor to treat the myeloma. A gal who is now a dear friend of mine and lives up the road from me said her husband had multiple myeloma and they thought his doctor was superior. Even though it is a two-and-a-half-hour drive each way to the cancer center, I do it gladly. You have to be willing to make extra effort to get extra-good care.

Over the years I have been on the receiving end of a lot of dismissive conversations from folks in the medical professions. During all this, one doctor actually said, "She is a hysterical female; give her some antidepressants."

I came through all this knowing that you have to have the courage of your convictions. You have to know yourself, and if you feel something is not right, act on that feeling and be willing to take an unpopular stand. That's not an easy thing to do, whether it concerns your health, employment, or personal relationships. You have to have the backbone to say, "It doesn't matter if other people think I am wrong or discount me." If you believe that what you are feeling is accurate, then act on it.

Documenting Your Journey

In this and subsequent chapters, we are going to suggest that you write things down as you take action to be at the center of your healthcare journey. This can be in a notebook, in an electronic document, using an online tool like CaringBridge (www.CaringBridge.org)—whatever works for you. Separately, you might also want to keep a journal to record your emotional experiences. We found that journaling helped us with the emotions and disorientation that come with a serious health journey. But, separate from a journal, the notebook/guide was very helpful; in fact, looking back, we wish we had done more with this tool, and that is reflected in our recommendations. Because of that, we are recommending a strong "take action" approach, but no one should feel they need to do everything we recommend. Do what is right for you.

Tip: Even if you're not into formal journaling, read through the four journaling steps outlined below—they will get you thinking about the important issues that you will face going forward and how to handle them. Then, if you want a quicker but still reliable record of your medical and emotional processes, take a look at the multiple checklists in Chapter 7. They help you set up everything from a record of your doctors' names and contact information to a wish list of your plans post-recovery.

Start Your Record of Your Journey

Step 1: Write what you understand your health situation to be, acknowledging that you are at the center of it. This description doesn't have to be complex or precise; just explain it in your own terms. Something happens when you put pen to paper or type words onto a screen. It is not enough to keep these thoughts in your head. The process of writing forces you to think and rethink your thoughts until they become increasingly clear. A clear written description might also help you communicate with clarity to members of your village and your care team.

Step 2: Write down your fears. Inventory them and perhaps rank them. Be honest. You have nothing to lose. This can be a private document or something shared with others. Don't worry about the potential judgments of others—that is their issue. If there is ever a time to be self-reflective and transparent in life, it is now.

Step 3: Write down your intentions for your journey, drawing on the sense of honesty that comes from doing steps 1 and 2. What do you expect to happen? When the going gets really tough, what intentions do you want to hold on to? There are some health journeys without a happy ending: diseases that are terminal or conditions that cause permanent impairment. You might want to express a sense of hope against even the hardest odds or describe your understanding of the limits you want to put on your treatments. But everyone, regardless of the length of their journeys or the likelihood of a particular outcome, deserves to have a journey in which they hold on to their integrity, their identity, and their humanity.

Think of your best self—the person you are on your best day, with the greatest sense of strength and clarity—and write what this best-self version of yourself would be during this health journey. By best self, we don't mean a miraculously flawless being; we mean a version of you that you'd be proud of even through the toughest journey. If it works for you and is important to you, don't be afraid to also write what you hope and dream and strive and pray for—the best outcome that you think is achievable. But the real goal is to write your intentions for yourself regardless of the odds, regardless of how hard things get, regardless of what other people think. What is the best self that you want to be? For Ed, his best self was to focus on resiliency. For Cris, his best self was to be as human as he could be under dehumanizing conditions.

Regardless of whether you approach your health journey as a fighter, an observer, or a participant, framing and documenting your intentions is critical. We have no judgment about which stance is best during a health journey. But we do believe that being an object without intention is a terrible way to endure a health journey.

Step 4: Write what you need to do, and what you need from others, to live the best-self version of your health journey. Again, be honest and do not worry who might read what you write. You need to lay everything on the table. Baring your soul is part of a more healthful journey.

This chapter comes with plenty of homework. Doing the homework may feel hard when you're on a significant health journey, but the resulting clarity and focus are worth it.

Now that you have accepted your own responsibility for your health journey, contemplated resilience, and gained better awareness, other realities will set in. This is where the value of the village can help you carry the weight. You need to develop a broader plan for your life today and in the future, whatever that may hold. Part 2 of this book will show you how.

Part Two

Making Your Healthcare Experience the Best It Can Be

A ll health journeys begin with you, but they are best not taken alone.

Surrounding you is your village. This includes family, friends, co-workers, maybe a support group of other people who share the same diagnosis. We know from research that engagement of families and friends to help a loved one through a health journey leads to better health outcomes and a better healthcare experience. And we know vividly from our own health experiences how much we relied on our villages. Ed's approach is formal and extensive; Cris's less so. Both approaches provided support that was appropriate, needed, and appreciated. Having support is not a nice-to-have, it's a must-have.

You might call it your village, team, gang, tribe, people, whatever! But no matter what they are to you, they are to be nurtured and never taken for granted.

We want to thank you for the privilege of being part of your village as you read this book and as you carry some of the ideas and to-dos with you through your journey.

—Ed and Cris

Five

It Takes a Village

How to create yours

How do you get the village that you deserve to support you through your healthcare journey?

The starting place is whomever you turn to today for connection and support in your moments of need. For instance, when you need help moving from one place to the next, who are the people who show up? Your village. Who is quick to defend you from accusations or the first to highlight your accomplishments? Who sends you texts or cards of support, love, and affirmation? Who reaches out to you looking for advice and feedback? Who makes you laugh? Whom do you run, swim, bike, or walk with?

However, the relationship between patient and village can be one of the most complex aspects of managing a serious health condition. Family and friends will inevitably have their own reactions, judgments, and opinions about your health. They may worry, feel anxious, say foolish or awkward things, or even object to how you are behaving. They may think, *My loved one isn't approaching their care correctly and should have a different attitude!* Sometimes the individuals you expect to be the most engaged with you during a crisis are the very ones who disappear. So give considerable thought to the people you choose to surround yourself with. Frequently, friends and family want to help but have no idea how. Like you, each member of your village has his or her own emotional reactions and experiences that they bring to your health journey.

In a way, you and your village pick each other. Sometimes the arrival of a difficult health journey can cause serious stress in relationships, and you may be surprised—pleasantly or unpleasantly—by people's reactions. We know patients who thought their family or partner was their village. However, when a crisis hit them, their family or partner was missing in action. We know of others who were overwhelmed with gratitude for a village that showed up out of nowhere. You may find that a person on the periphery turns out to be a solid and invaluable supporter during your crisis. Perhaps the only predictable thing about how your potential village will respond to your health crisis is that it is unpredictable.

There are lots of ways people live in their villages before, during, and after a health crisis. Ed's village was large and boisterous, a wide circle of friends and supporters. He was in frequent communication with and in the presence of this supportive group. Cris's village was small and closely held: daughters, girlfriend, and a few close friends and neighbors. He maintained communication with others via emails and an online patient support app, CaringBridge. He often found it difficult to ask for help but was very grateful for the help he received.

You may be somewhere between Cris's and Ed's styles, or you might be even more private or more outgoing. But everyone needs help—as CaringBridge says, "no one should go through a health journey alone."

Approaches to Your Village

If you picked up this book because you or a loved one is facing a health crisis, you will want to rally a village in whatever ways you can. There are many kinds of villages. Some villages are created during a health crisis and are impromptu. You do the best you can in the situation. We give you some pointers on how to make these villages as effective as possible.

Some villages may be nothing more than a single friend who is with you helping however they can. No formalities. No structure. But they are there for you.

Some villages may be what we call a quiet village, a small group of existing family or friends with whom you are already connected and who rally around you.

Some villages will be more formal. They will have structure, such as routine meetings. Often these are built on existing social structures such as an affinity group or a faith-related group.

We will share best practices to strengthen these common manifestations of villages.

The Impromptu Village

This village is created in the midst of crisis. While you may be tempted to skip the curation of a village, we encourage you to try your best to make one happen. You may feel exhausted, stressed, and anxious, but an impromptu village will help you in many important ways. Reach out to family and friends you think might be of help and lean on them. Ask for immediate help. You deserve it. Your journey will be better for having this support.

Later, your impromptu village may evolve into something more structured. For example, a group of friends from your children's school may set up a system to get your kids to soccer games and piano lessons while you are hospitalized or receiving treatment. As time allows, you and your impromptu village may find that you naturally improve your communication, and the village members increase the support they provide.

The Quiet Village and the Challenges of Asking for Help

If you are a person who is most comfortable with a quiet village, you know who you want in your circle. It can be surprising or disappointing to find out that your village didn't rally as you had hoped. Having someone disappear or be unable to help you is more noticeable. Please remember that someone failing to show up is probably because of some real challenge that your friend faces and is not about you or your relationship with them. Maybe a loved one in their life died of the disease that you've been diagnosed with, and they just can't face it again. Maybe they care about you deeply but can't face being with you when you're sick. Maybe they have some deep-seated phobia around healthcare or are squeamish about being around illness. Who knows? Be grateful for the people who can show up, and as you go through and emerge from your illness do whatever you need to do to repair your relationships with the people who can't or don't show up.

> *Cris's **quiet village:** I am blessed to have wonderful daughters, a calm and wise girlfriend, and a wide circle of great friends and supportive neighbors. My village of professional colleagues is large and extended. I'm an extrovert who loves being out and about with friends, going places and doing things, and in my business life I am in touch with hundreds of people daily. I get energy*

from crowds, people, and activity. But when it comes to health, I'm an introvert and I have trouble asking for help. When I went through cancer—and then shortly thereafter had to help my mom through her illness and death—I circled the wagons. For me, a more private and intimate support group is exactly what I needed. My healthcare village was my daughters, my girlfriend, and close friends who volunteered to do specific things for me. I also connected with fellow travelers—I think of my cancer buddy John, a priest from Pennsylvania, who always had radiation therapy on the same day as me. We both rang the end-of-radiation bell on the same day. He was a temporary but important member of my village. I also found out that not everyone could or would join me on my journey. I think of a dear friend who contacted me immediately after my first diagnosis and expressed her sadness, but also said, "I'm not good in crises. I can be a friend, but I know I won't be of much help. I'll see you on the other side." I treasured her honesty and knew that her response was colored by past family health crises. She was off the hook and is still a dear friend.

For those of you who find it difficult to ask for help, a couple of things you might consider:

- First, remind yourself that having a village is necessary for a successful health journey, and you deserve it. Those who prefer a quiet village might feel guilty asking for help or might feel that asking for help will create uncomfortable obligations. Those feelings are probably illusory; most people really do want to help someone they care about. You matter, and this is a significant situation. Just press on and ask for help, even if it's uncomfortable.

- Second, consider using digital means for connection—the tool of choice for introverts and millennials. Cris is on the board of directors of CaringBridge, which is a free online tool for patients and their caregivers to share information with friends and family about the patient's health journey and for helping friends and family coordinate care for a patient or their loved ones as they go through difficult times. It can also serve as a place to express feelings and document a difficult journey. It's a great tool to communicate confidentially with your village. In addition, it has built-in ways to ask people for help, with request lists, calendars, and other tools. Cris used the app throughout his second healthcare journey, posting brief written updates, which were especially helpful in communicating with the broader circle of friends who cared about him and wanted to know what was going on, even if they were not part of the intimate village caring for him. There are many online digital communities you can tap into for support. Mayo Clinic has communities open to everyone, not just Mayo patients; the program is called Mayo Clinic Connect (https://connect .mayoclinic.org). Other hospitals and disease-specific support groups have similar online resources to help you learn about your diagnosis, chosen treatments and their consequences, and their impact on your daily life.

- Third, consider taking advantage of villages that already exist. We highly recommend plugging into any resources provided by your healthcare organization, disease-related support groups, and community support groups. They can be digital, as we just described, or in-person support groups.

- Many workplaces have formal groups organized around wellness and illness, such as weight-loss groups, yoga, or other exercise groups and even disease support groups for patients, to name a few. Even in the new world of remote and hybrid work, a village organized around your workplace can be convenient because of location, shared experience, and context, which can help you bond with other members. Obviously, privacy can be a challenge if you're opening up to coworkers, but it may be worth it to you.

- Patient advocacy groups are another opportunity to use already existing villages in order to build your own. Many times your local healthcare organization will establish these. These groups exist online and in person. Ed is on the board of the North Texas Prostate Cancer Coalition. All board members are men who have battled prostate cancer, and together they created educational content and the support framework and foundations for villages to happen. Ed can attest that over the years they have been the village for many men who have been diagnosed with prostate cancer.

- There are also patient advocates you can hire. They are paid to be part of your village (or, in extreme cases, your entire village). Just as you might hire a nurse to take care of you or a loved one at home, you can do something similar by hiring a patient advocate. These arrangements range from full-time advocacy, in which the advocate attends your clinical visits and helps process your medical bills, to part-time advocacy, which lets you pick up the phone and ask questions or receive support as you need it. Board-certified patient advocates (BCPAs) are the highest-credentialed professional patient advocates; they support patients' and families' unmet needs while protecting their rights and ensuring that care is aligned with personal goals and values. Just as an example, Enlightening Results, founded by Grace Cordovano, Ph.D., BCPA, is an example of a private patient advocacy practice specializing in oncology. Enlightening Results assists patients with a cancer diagnosis while navigating the complex US healthcare system.

The Structured Village

A structured village is one that you intentionally set out to form, and it calls for routine care for friends and family—and for their care for you—so that you can all acknowledge your interdependence in both good times and bad. You may form it, as Ed and Simran have, because of your deep belief in the emotional and physical benefits of close ties and shared responsibility for one another.

That belief motivated them to establish a village after Ed experienced the "widowmaker" and before his cancer diagnosis. They didn't know it would be needed for another health crisis—but it certainly was a source of great support and comfort when that second diagnosis happened.

If you embrace the concept of a structured village, you may establish it before a health crisis strikes or during a health crisis and you want to continue to nurture it when that health crisis is over. So keep in mind the following two points, which help establish and reinforce its structure and integrity.

- **Routine.** Structured villages require consistency. You should establish a routine cadence. The maximum amount of time that should go by without a formal touch point is a month. Always remember that time is a gift—and a limited one. Most people are willing to commit an hour at a time, but when they are asked for more, their commitment can dim. A weekly two-hour meeting might sound great to you, but short, action-packed meetings once or twice a month are better than long meetings every week that have members questioning the value of participating.

- **Diversity.** As in all other aspects of life, the more diverse and inclusive the village, the stronger it is. When everyone is the same, you get the same. When there is a mix of different cultures, races, religions, and ethnicities, you get a more comprehensive blend of ideas and help and skills. We look forward to the day—and hope it is soon—when all villages are blended and can draw on the strength gained from diversity in all its manifestations.

For those interested in developing a more structured village:

- Take a few moments to write out a list of the people in your village or whom you might like in your village.
- Bounce your list off a partner, spouse, or best friend for additional insights.

- The process of thinking deeply about your village and writing names will help crystallize these critical relationships. With the list in hand, you should be proactive in nurturing these relationships—hopefully before you need them again.

Ed and Simran's village life: Simran and I understand the power of a village, but a few years ago we realized we were lacking when it came to having strong, like-minded married couples in our lives. One evening we sat down and talked about other couples we knew whom we admired and who could complement and support our marital journey. We desired a racially and ethnically diverse set of couples who would battle for one another and with whom we could just be gut honest about life and love and death. The "Texas Ten" was born—Texas because this is where we live, and ten because we were five couples. We went to each couple and explained how we desired to be surrounded by other couples who would all commit to the relationships long-term through routine interactions and gut-honest communications. One couple was lukewarm, and we moved past them. We reasoned that if they needed to be convinced of the value of such a group, they would always need pushing and prodding. Everyone else was enthusiastic. We consist of Christians, atheists, and Hindus. We are from different racial backgrounds. We were born in Germany, China, India, Nigeria, and the United States. We are beautiful and wonderfully made. A cultural kaleidoscope.

The Texas Ten has been going strong since late 2019. As a group, we met in person one time prior to the pandemic. Throughout 2020 and most of 2021, we met every other Saturday over Zoom.

The requirements were: you must have something to drink, make 90 percent of the meetings, and be fully engaged. To accelerate the discovery process we went deep and provocative in each meeting on heavy topics such as race, trauma, mistakes, and death. We gave one another the gift of time, where each person shared their story uninterrupted. Oh, so many tears of loss, but also tears of joy. With each meeting we grew closer and more liberated as people. I am convinced that any member of the Texas Ten would give their life for another. They are a key part of our village. The village concept, and the Texas Ten specifically, is so powerful we have others asking to join! We recently expanded to another couple, who reside in the neighboring state of Oklahoma. They routinely drive into Texas to meet with us and celebrate milestones of all kinds. We consider ourselves lucky to have developed this village before my second health crisis.

You can do something similar. For us, we wanted to form a group with other married couples. But your village can be a village of painters, or even a village of wine connoisseurs (as described below). It can be members of a church, mosque, or synagogue. It can be a subset of leaders from work. Be creative. The key is to take action now. If you are into a specific hobby or sport, start there.

Ed recalls: *We have a friend who loves wine. He joined an existing village of eclectic individuals who had their own private speakeasy inside a nondescript warehouse. The speakeasy contained a secured, temperature-controlled vault for storing extensive wine collections. Members would drop in on weekends and sit in one of the living rooms and share their favorite wines. Over months and years,* *relationships were formed and forged. When someone encountered challenging circumstances, members would surround that person with love and support.*

We have relatives who are transgender. Given societal and family pressures, it was critical for them to find a village inside the LGBTQ+ community who could directly relate to their unique challenges. In this village they found strength and resolve and acceptance.

Once you create a strong village, consider expanding outside the boundaries of your community and engage others who might add value and help. The more diverse your village, the stronger your support system becomes.

The workplace also provides ample opportunities to find or develop your village. We know clinicians who not only love taking care of patients but love technology as well. They formed a society where they meet regularly, share a meal, and listen to a peer present on ideas at the intersection of technology and clinical science. Because of the routine of gathering and sharing meals and because of the vulnerability involved in standing and sharing before peers, relationships are born and cultivated and expanded. Some of these individuals will likely rally around any member of the group in time of need.

When Ed's health crises hit, the already-formed village was a great help. But he also discovered that his village included surprise members.

Ed: *Shortly after I went public with my cancer diagnosis, I returned to my office. The Cleveland Clinic culture extends into* *everything, including office decor and furnishings. Everything is color-coordinated, and there is no deviation. Some might call it modern; I found it sterile but functional. But the emotional "decor" is vivid, colorful, and downright beautiful. My colleagues are part of my village—just as my family and friends are.*

Two weeks prior to my surgery, many of my closest friends met up at one of their houses and we partied hard. We poured Stag's Leap, my favorite vineyard. At the end of the night, they all laid hands on me and prayed for healing. I felt loved.

One week prior we had our annual family reunion. At the end, a handful of nieces and nephews, brothers and sisters, and sons and daughters did the same—they laid hands on me, speaking words of love and blessing. I gained confidence knowing so many people had my back and my family's too.

Then . . . imagine my surprise when I walked into my office a few days prior to my surgery and the walls were covered in brightly colored four-leaf clovers. Each leaf was uniquely decorated with well-wishes from members of the information technology department. I had been going through a mix of emotions as I grappled with cancer, and this act of love felt overwhelmingly good. My work colleagues had my back. I read each one and gave thanks for all the thoughts and prayers these represented. I kept every one of these, and after my recovery I created a mosaic from the leaves.

Cancer had nothing on me! I had my village!

Ed's village redux: *On the one-year anniversary of my widow-maker, my wife, Simran, organized a surprise party. I was asked* *to dress in a tuxedo with a red bow tie and to be prepared for a fantastic evening. We love to go out and party, so I did not think too much about what was going on . . . until I was blindfolded. I was escorted into a banquet hall, where one of my sons removed my eye covering. Surprise! The hall was filled with members of my village from all around the country, each person's outfit accented in red. There were family, coworkers, Team USA teammates, close friends, and, yes, even those who may be on the fringes but who are always there in a crisis. I still tear up as I write in remembrance of that fabulous evening.*

Here's one more powerful example of a village that incorporates many of the ideas above.

Ed's first village: I will admit this village was created before I knew what a village was, but I am glad we were a part of it! In 1993 our oldest daughter was born. Despite inducements, my wife's womb refused to release the gift inside. I went from coach to frightened bystander. Finding my way behind Simran, I stroked her hair and whispered prayers in her ear. The delivery room filled quickly with physicians and nurses we didn't recognize. Walls shifted to reveal medical equipment, completing the transition from birthing suite to operating theater.

I kept one eye on the fetal heart monitor. Fluctuating wildly, the bottom fell out. Flatline. Seconds passed but seemed like minutes. After cutting, vacuuming, forceps, and manipulation, our baby appeared. "We've got a floppy," someone called. The doctor handed her to the nurse. Resuscitation began.

Seven minutes later, the nurse lifted our now-breathing child and said, "Here's your daughter," even as they made their way toward the newborn intensive care unit (NICU).

In the NICU, Talitha slept in isolation. We could look but not touch. She was fighting multiple afflictions. Physicians forecasted grim physical and mental damage. I left the hospital that morning around 3 a.m. My wife remained hospitalized with severe trauma to her body given the efforts to deliver our daughter. I slept for two or three hours and then got my son ready for school. I headed back to the hospital to check in on my wife and daughter. When I walked into her room, I was shocked to see twenty people there, all members of a small group we belonged to at our local church. They were essentially our village.

The village took over. They arranged meals for thirty days. They arranged transportation for our son to get to school and back. This was truly a godsend. We could now focus on my wife's and daughter's healing. Frankly, I don't know if we would have survived without the village. Eight days later, Talitha was released from the hospital, and she suffered no long-term physical or mental damage. She graduated from college at eighteen and serves in healthcare today. My wife fully recovered as well.

The Village in Marginalized Communities

The village is especially important in marginalized communities where lack of access to healthcare, scant economic resources, and systemic prejudices mean that each patient needs as much emotional support and as many advocates as possible. Your village can help you fight for the care you need and help keep an eye out for slights and oversights that need to be called out and overcome. In certain communities, such as the LGBTQ+ community, some members may be cut off from family and the broader community. Both of us have family or friends who are transgender. Cris has spent time supporting unhoused and refugee families. We acknowledge how hard it can be to create or maintain a village of support when someone comes from a marginalized community, or simply where family ties may be strained or broken, or where community connections and resources are thin. With respect, we believe that every person deserves a village. For people who face discrimination or isolation, our prayer is that you will not hide or be shamed or be fearful of approaching a village or creating one. For people who live in remote areas or identify as part of a marginalized community, online resources can be a lifeline, providing a virtual village of support.

> *Ed: One of my nephews transitioned and is now my niece. I watched and supported the transition carefully, both as a family member and as a healthcare executive. At the time of this writing, there remain some communities, like LGBTQ+ in general and transgender specifically, who remain somewhat alienated from healthcare systems. Rural residents, people of color, and those with reduced financial resources are also often shortchanged in the quality of care they have and their ability to fight for the care they need.*

Keeping Your Village Strong

Embracing the Process

Creating a village of any kind—impromptu, quiet, or structured—is not a onetime event. You should continuously build your village. You will meet people in the course of your healthcare journey who might become part of your village or lead you to others who may be of help.

You may want to become part of another patient's village. To the extent you are able, give your time to another patient. Doing so not only will help them; it may give you more ideas about how to grow or enhance your own village. You may meet new friends. And you may discover resources that will help you as well. Sometimes when we give to others it is we who receive the most.

There are a few things you can do to nurture a sense of village.

- **Leadership.** You may need to be the leader in the beginning, when you are initially reaching out to people for help, but don't feel like you need to be in charge of the village all the way through. There may be trusted people you can ask to take the lead. You might turn to your spouse or a family member or friend to coordinate the activities of your village. You could also be a little more structured and ask for different people to take a turn coordinating your village.
- **Partnership.** If there is no existing village and you want to create one, reach out to one other person to partner with you. They can help carry the load. There is nothing wrong with asking for help and co-leading. This is especially important if your health situation is overwhelming. A partner can take responsibility for gatherings, organize support you might need, and expand the village if needed.
- **Engagement.** You need to do more than just show up. You must be fully present. Your village will follow your lead. While you do not want to make membership onerous, you should

have a few standards that help with engagement. Examples include no phones out at the meetings and no multitasking. It can be deflating when you are discussing serious health matters and there are secondary conversations taking place or social media–related distractions. This does mean that you need to be organized and use the available time smartly.

- **Vulnerability.** When you are transparent with your feelings and your life, it invites empathy and helps your village members have a clearer idea about how you are feeling and what you may need. Do not withhold emotions. If you need to curse, then curse. If you need to cry, then cry. Your vulnerability will create the doorway for others to follow; connections begin and your village unfolds. If you are stoic and everything in your life appears perfect, your village will have a harder time offering you effective support.

- **Communication.** Communication is the lifeblood of any community, and your village is no different. Communication can be as simple as email. The key is routine communication but not spam. You want to be careful not to email too much, but at the same time, you need to find the right balance that keeps the village informed and engaged. The Texas Ten find that the WhatsApp platform seems to work best for them; it is pretty easy to post things and keep the village updated while sharing pictures and videos.

Actions That All Villages Can Take

There is a wide range of supports and services that a village can provide. As you put together your team, think about what you may want them to do for you and talk to each member about what kinds of help you may need from them.

When someone falls ill, they may need assistance in one or all of the following areas. They include attending to everyday needs and tasks as well as managing important areas involving finance, insurance, employment, and technology-based "paperwork" that needs to be taken care of.

- **Childcare.** For those with kids still at home, helping out might include getting kids to and from school, providing care or other support after school, helping with homework, and so on. If the kids are teenagers, don't assume they are self-sufficient; checking in on their mental health is especially critical.
- **Pets.** One element that you might not think of when you build your village is pets. Dogs, cats, horses, and even tropical fish are important village members, providing solace, love, and amusement. But they also need TLC. They will miss you when you're in the hospital or otherwise unable to care for them, and they need to be tended to by other village members.
- **Groceries.** Depending on the situation, help with groceries may be needed. Sometimes the act of shopping requires too much energy, and in that case shopping for someone can alleviate significant stress.
- **Meals.** It is pretty easy to develop a routine for the village to provide meals for the impacted family. When this responsibility is rotated, the burden is light for the village but the support for the patient is significant.
- **Bills.** Sometimes it is the routine things of life that most often are neglected when someone is in crisis. Bill paying is

one of those areas. Perhaps someone can be assigned to look at inbound email and postal mail and ensure that all bills are processed. There is nothing worse than dealing with your health crisis and suddenly finding that debt collectors are calling and threatening to turn off needed services.

- **Surprises.** If the village can do it, surprise your friend with blessings big and small. Take a look at their car. Is it in need of repair or routine maintenance or even just a tankful of gas? You can hire a cleaning service or arrange for a cleaning day when the village comes over to scrub down the house or take care of the yard. Even the smallest of gestures will have a huge impact on those who are sick.

- **Clothing and personal services.** Even when someone is hospitalized, new clothes or towels might make the hospital stay a little better. The same is true if someone is convalescing at home. There is nothing like a pedi or mani or even a haircut to make you feel better.

- **Insurance.** Ensure that someone establishes communications with your health insurance as needed so that nothing falls through the cracks. You want them to collect and organize the "explanations of benefits" you will receive in the mail or electronically. The last thing you need to fret about during your journey is insurance.

- **Work schedule.** If you're employed, you may want a village member (who also might be a coworker) to keep your manager in the loop about how you are doing and when you might be back to work.

- **Transportation.** How will you get to and from all your appointments? You want a primary person as well as a backup person to be available. Even so, there may be times when people you count on have to work or are out of town. Have your transportation provider work with you to identify ride services you can access when needed. Many hospitals now have special programs to help you with transportation.

- **Communication within the village.** Your village members may be in different locations, may not know each other well, or may not be in communication with one another very often. If that's the case, you might designate someone to have the specific role of making sure all village members know about developments in your condition and are aware as new needs arise.

- **Health system technology.** Many health systems offer digital tools for patients, and it can be daunting—but if you need assistance, someone in your village may be able to help you interact with your hospital's and/or doctor's digital app so that you can get into your patient portal. This will streamline communication with clinicians and help you manage all aspects of healthcare, from medications and appointments to test results.

- **Critical family documents.** Some health journeys are serious enough that you or the loved one you are caring for loses their healthcare battle. If so, having an advance directive, a medical power of attorney, a will, and an executor for the estate will make life easier. Store critical documents like wills and advance

ADVANCE DIRECTIVES

An advance directive not only means that you will get the care that you want—do you want to be resuscitated? Do you want extraordinary efforts taken to keep you alive?—but also reduces the stress and pain for your family and others if you are unable to make medical decisions or are approaching death. Make sure this form is embedded in your electronic health record and that all clinicians are aware of your wishes.

> *Ed: When my mom was dying of ovarian cancer, I had her create an advance directive so that there would be no question about how I would handle end-of-life matters for her. The trauma of her passing was tough enough on our family, so being able to follow her blueprint for dying and how she wanted her funeral arranged gave me significant peace and provided unity for our family.*

The directive typically covers five questions regarding how you want your care handled should you become incapacitated:

1. Whom you want to make healthcare decisions for you when you can't make them.
2. The kind of medical treatment you want or don't want.
3. How comfortable you want to be.
4. How you want people to treat you.
5. What you want your loved ones to know.

healthcare directives in a safe place and make sure family members know where they are.

Keeping Your Village Together During Your Health Crisis

Though the purpose of your village is to support you, paradoxically your other job may be to attend to the well-being of those in your village. One of your primary roles as the patient is to help ensure that members are comfortable being on your team.

While those in your village are genuinely interested in being on your team, when a health crisis arises members will feel a mix of fear, enthusiasm, and ignorance. You can't assume that everyone understands your medical situation. Some may have questions but be afraid to ask them, because they may be afraid of offending you or appearing inept. You will need to go out of your way to ensure that those in your village can ask questions, that their questions are answered, and that they understand your hopes and expectations. You might consider bringing your village together virtually or physically so that you can tell them collectively about your situation and invite questions.

No Rubber Stamp: Confrontation, Love, New Understandings

The role of the village is not all butterflies and roses. At times it may be important for them to challenge you.

> *Ed: I recall driving with Cris from the Twin Cities to Rochester to accompany him to some medical appointments at Mayo Clinic. Cris explained that one of his goals was to avoid having an ostomy. Cris had told his surgical team that this was his priority and that he was willing to accept a higher chance of cancer recurrence from*

> *a less aggressive surgery if that meant preserving enough of his*
> *digestive system so that he could avoid the ostomy. I challenged*
> *Cris because I didn't want my friend to die! Cris explained his*
> *reasoning, and after I pushed him a few times, I knew his decision*
> *was not just an emotional one but based on sound thinking about*
> *what was best for him.*

Your village is empowered to challenge you even if it makes you upset. Support, like love, can sometimes come in the way of a challenge. And you are empowered to push back and to express your point of view clearly and with passion. After all, it is your illness. Everyone in the village needs to know this up front.

Action Step: Create a Village

This chapter and the next chapter, on putting together your care team, end with action steps. The elements of these steps are what we suggest, but feel free to adjust each element based on your personal preferences and comfort level.

Brainstorm

Take a few minutes and think about relationships and communities where you are connected. Write out the names of the people who you believe would be there for you in a health crisis. Don't be too picky here; just have a free flow of ideas. Perhaps invite a friend or partner to help you. Consider people at your workplace, family members and friends, and people in any other communities you participate in (such as a religious community or hobby community).

Identify Village Members

From your brainstormed list of people who you think would be there for you in a crisis, create a list of people you might want in your village. Be aware that this list may change over time.

We know from our own experiences and from research that many people have a very hard time asking for help. Our experience was that almost everyone close to us wanted to help and was happy to be asked. Many volunteered what they wanted to do for us and communicated how they wanted to be with us through our journeys. Some wanted to help but didn't know how; they welcomed being asked to do specific things. Some couldn't help with the things we asked for but offered to help in other useful ways, some of which we hadn't considered. And some people, we found, had a hard time following through, usually because of other demands in their lives or because they had difficulty being with us when we were seriously ill.

Join an Existing Village

Earlier in this chapter we wrote about patient support groups, advocacy groups, and other resources. You might consider how you could engage with such groups as part of your village.

Add the Village to Your Notebook or Journal

Here's an example of how you might list your potential or actual village team members and their roles. This is for someone we have named Tim.

- *Susan.* Patient partner/co-leader. Her role: Be supportive of Tim. Assist him.

- *Gerry.* Village manager. His role: Check in on Tim and Susan. Ensure that the village meets regularly and that Tim and Susan are getting full support.
- *Angela.* Village administrator. Her role: Schedule meetings. Make sure we do everything we agree to do.
- *Jacob.* Rabbi. His role: Ensure the spiritual wellness of the village.
- *Rachael.* Village member and Tim and Susan's neighbor. Her role: Available to help with transportation or food prep.
- *Fran.* Tim's coworker. Their role: Liaison with work on issues such as benefits and remote work.
- *Brian.* Tim's brother. His role: Brother stuff.
- *Esther.* Tim's sister. Her role: Sister stuff.

In addition to names and roles, you might want to jot down attitudes you want to embrace or things you want to say to village members, such as:

- Please listen to me when I need to share something.
- Please be present in whatever ways work for you.
- Understand it is hard for me to ask for help.

None of this is set in stone. Feel free to experiment with styles and formats, and find what kind of village works best for you. It's not what your village looks like; it's that you have one for the journey.

Six

Putting Together Your Care Team

Your journey begins with you, and hopefully you have the right village supporting you. But you also will be surrounded by, guided by, and supported by your care team. Your care team is made up of everyone who provides medical and supportive care. It includes facilities such as the hospitals and clinics where you receive care. But because your healthcare journey begins with you, we believe that you, and not a clinician, should be the center of your care team.

That may be a challenging idea. Many people want to defer to their doctor or don't feel like they have the knowledge or ability to be at the center. But you can do it, and you should do it to the degree you are willing and able.

When putting your care team together, you want to be engaged in deciding where you get treated, who is on your care team, how your care team functions, and what medical decisions it makes. Your care team works *with* you to create a treatment plan, define your path, and establish goals for care. To the greatest extent possible, given your circumstances:

- You should be active in deciding who is going to care for you.
- You should be intentional about your journey, using whatever tools and approaches you feel are right for you as you put your care team together.
- You should stay engaged in the ongoing management of your care team.

In short, this is where the rubber meets the road!

When You Have to Battle to Find the Right Care Team

This chapter describes steps in assembling your best care team, and at first glance they may seem like some easy-to-get-through items that can lead you gracefully and inevitably to your best outcome. But we know that they are far from easy. No story so clearly demonstrates how engaged and aggressive you need to be to get the care you deserve than Debra's.

Debra: I have worked in healthcare for over forty years, and I was married to a doctor, but I fell through the cracks with convoluted misdiagnoses over and over from a well-respected local cardiologist. I sought a second opinion outside my area, and that physician added additional information that also proved wrong.

I was first diagnosed with a mitral valve prolapse, then aortic stenosis, then small blood vessel disease, and finally subaortic membrane, and I was told by my local cardiologist I needed to have open heart surgery and the local heart surgeon could perform it. In the end, what I truly was contending with was hypertrophic obstructive cardiomyopathy and, eventually, heart failure. I can only imagine what would have happened had I proceeded with open heart surgery for a diagnosis I did not have!

Over several years, I knew I was getting worse. I couldn't run. I could barely hike anymore, and I was no longer able to walk fast. One time I remember stopping at least fourteen times in less than two miles. But I had trust in my medical community. And during this time my (adoptive) mom and dad were both extremely ill and needed my care, so I pushed aside my concerns to focus on them.

I was so stressed that two days after my mom died, I went to my primary care physician. He listened to my heart and immediately sent me back to the cardiologist for an echocardiogram.

The cardiologist misdiagnosed me once again with a pretty rare congenital condition called subaortic membrane, which would require open heart surgery. He assured me, one more time, that the local heart surgeon could perform this surgery.

I was hesitant to go forward, especially since he said this was so rare and I wondered how many such surgeries the recommended doctor had performed. So I did my research and learned what a center of excellence is. I knew such care was not available locally, so I decided on two outstanding places to go for cardiac issues and asked to be referred to Cedars-Sinai in L.A. and Mayo Clinic in Rochester. Neither was close by!

I first went to Cedars-Sinai and three months later Mayo Clinic in Rochester. Both places were able to accurately diagnose what I actually had: hypertrophic obstructive cardiomyopathy. But Mayo had the approach I liked—even though it scared me when Dr. Evans said I should not ride my motorcycle, because of the risk of SCD [sudden cardiac death]. He said it could happen at any time, but especially during stressful situations or extreme exertion. Because of this he also said not to lift weights or even do yoga—which no one else had mentioned. I had been doing that all along, and it could have killed me! Who knew? Not me!

It was the visit to Mayo the made all the difference and helped me make my decision. They ordered two simple tests that no doctor had done before: a BNP lab test and a chest X-ray. The results showed I was developing heart failure. Why somebody had not done these tests before is beyond me. And how about a simple chest X-ray? My heart was enlarged and extended down below my diaphragm.

I have learned my case isn't uncommon. I am not sure of the actual statistics, but a large percentage of folks with hypertrophic obstructive cardiomyopathy are not diagnosed promptly. The doctors don't see it in their everyday practice, and because this is not common, they treat symptoms, not causes, and don't go looking for anything outside garden-variety heart disease. So my advice is, don't be rushed through appointments and be sure you are heard. And listen to your body. You know how you feel, and you know when something is wrong, and sometimes you need to educate your doctor.

Today, after a septal myectomy at Mayo, Rochester, I am feeling so much better. I have my life back! I can walk, I don't get chest pain, I no longer gasp for air, nor have terrible exhaustion. I am back in the swing of things, regularly taking four-to-six-mile walks and enjoying the blessings of life. I got a second chance because even though I am not assertive, I knew I had to be my own advocate, and I am so grateful I was.

Making the Choices That Are Right for You

We recognize that, depending on your situation and your particular circumstances, your range of choices about where and by whom to be treated may be narrow or wide. Your choices may be determined by geography, insurance coverage, or other factors. In some cases, there may be only a handful of clinicians who can properly care for you and only one or two facilities that offer the care you need. But for many of you, you may have more choices than you think.

For us, our choices about where to be treated were pretty easy. Ed had a heart attack while running a duathlon, and the ambulance took him to the race-event-designated hospital equipped with a Level 1 (highest-level) trauma center. When Ed had prostate cancer, he knew he wanted to be treated at his hospital, Cleveland Clinic. When Cris had cancer, he knew he wanted to be treated at Mayo Clinic.

The choice about who would treat us was a little more complicated. Prior to Ed's prostatectomy, he interviewed two candidates who recommended materially different approaches to the surgery. One surgeon used an open technique, while the other leveraged a less invasive robotic approach. Ed opted for the surgeon adept at the open technique because of his existing trusted friendship with that physician.

Cris was referred to an oncologist and surgeon. Cris was lucky, as an insider, to be able to talk with the head of the colorectal surgical division. He offered to do Cris's surgery but said if it were his surgery or that of a loved one, he would use the surgeon to whom Cris was already referred. That made the choice easy. When Cris met his oncologist, he felt confident in him and felt they could communicate well. After treatment of his cancer, he needed to work with the right gastroenterologist to help manage aftercare. When the first one wasn't a great fit, he asked for help in getting one with more experience managing the aftereffects of his surgeries.

We acknowledge that it's a bit of a toss-up whether you should pick your clinicians or facility first. In Step 2 we address how to pick clinicians. In Step 3 we address how to pick a facility.

Because we believe that your journey begins with you, we recommend an activist approach in choosing your care team. But we understand that one size does not fit all. Each person will approach their healthcare journey and the assembly of their care team with a unique attitude. Our intent is to share models and approaches that you can adjust based on who you are and how you confront challenges and difficulties.

The activist approach we suggest might work for you. You may even want to go further than we suggest. Or you may want to take a less activist stance and delegate decisions to your care team or your village. That's all OK. Our view is that you should be as intentional as possible about your journey, using whatever tools and approaches are right for you. Just stay true to your intentions.

So to begin on this pathway of you managing your care, let's take a look at how you build your care team.

Step 1: Learn About Your Diagnosis and Options for Care

You should be purposeful in learning more about your condition. That will empower you. You should also prepare yourself for the fact that you might be frightened as you learn more. You may be angry, sad, depressed, scared. You might feel a sense of hope or optimism: *Maybe it's not as bad as I thought.* Or you might feel a sense of hopelessness and pessimism: *Maybe I can't do this.*

Understanding your condition can cause a whole stew of feelings—sometimes those feelings can come all at once, and often they may seem contradictory. Despite the intensity of these potential emotional reactions, we encourage you to research your condition or diagnosis. If you have a close member of your village whom you trust, they might feel capable of doing research for you and summarizing the key things to know. That can be a good way of buffering some of the potentially negative news and providing a balanced view. Regardless, it is important to know what you are fighting.

Knowing more makes it *your* journey, will help you be resilient, and will help you make important decisions about selecting and working with your care team.

Initially, you probably will get information and guidance from your primary care or diagnosing physician. This is one place where having a village helps. Most people have a hard time remembering and processing everything their clinician tells them, especially if the diagnosis is serious. Having someone come with you to appointments is very helpful. Your caregiver can listen, take notes and ask questions, and then afterward draw on those to fill in anything you may have missed or not fully processed. We'll address this in more detail in Step 6—Introducing Village Members to Your Care Team.

We suggest that you supplement what you learn from your clinicians with other, independent sources. We also believe that you should rely on authoritative sources. Especially during the COVID–19 pandemic, people looking for hope and people skeptical about Big Medicine or Big Pharma sometimes turned to sources that were naive, or motivated by philosophy or politics rather than science, and consequently were guided to questionable or dangerous treatments. It's best to depend on sources that are rooted in published research and authoritative organizations.

Some websites that can reliably help you learn more about your diagnosis include but are not limited to:

- CDC.gov
- MayoClinic.org
- my.clevelandclinic.org
- WebMD.com
- Internet sites specific to your disease, like the websites of the American Heart Association (www.heart.org) and the American Cancer Society (cancer.org)
- Disease-specific support groups
- Various academically oriented health systems (Cedars-Sinai, Mount Sinai, New York–Presbyterian/Columbia, Johns Hopkins, and many others)

Our suggestion that you rely on authoritative, independent sources of information does not mean you should necessarily limit your search to sources focusing on conventional medical care. There are also great authoritative sources devoted to alternative and complementary care, which are valid and important supplemental forms of treatment. Some websites that can reliably help you to learn more about alternative treatments and complementary medicine include but are not limited to:

- The National Center for Complementary and Integrative Health (www.nccih.nih.gov)
- Mayo Clinic (www.mayoclinic.org/departments-centers /integrative-medicine-health)
- Cleveland Clinic (my.clevelandclinic.org/departments/wellness /integrative)

- Websites sponsored by science-based disease-specific organizations, like:
  - ◦ The National Cancer Society site on complementary and alternative medicine (www.cancer.gov/about-cancer /treatment/cam)
  - ◦ The American Cancer Society site on alternative treatments (www.cancer.org/cancer/managing-cancer/treatment-types /alternative-medicine.html)

You may want to go farther afield and find different websites, books, and advocates. By all means keep an open mind, but be careful.

Finally, depending on your situation, you may feel that a new treatment may be appropriate for your condition. Many healthcare organizations, in particular academic medical centers associated with a university or medical school, participate in and provide clinical trials for eligible patients. Depending on the rarity or severity of your condition, you may come across clinical trials in your research about care options. The National Library of Medicine maintains a comprehensive catalog of all privately or publicly funded clinical trials around the world—hundreds of thousands of them—at www.clinicaltrials.gov. You can search the database by condition or location. At the beginning of your journey, it's probably too early to determine whether a clinical trial is right for you, but when you are researching providers and hospitals you may want to consider whether such trials are available with the providers or hospitals you are considering.

As you gain insights into your condition or diagnosis and next possible steps, it's time to begin choosing who will provide your medical care. We start with who will be on your care team (Step 2), but in some cases you will want or need to begin by choosing where you will receive care (Step 3). Think of them as a pair.

Step 2: Choosing Your Care Team Members

Too often, we relinquish control to clinicians, out of respect, out of fear, or from a belief this is the way it is supposed to be. After all, you think (or hope) the professionals are experienced with your specific disease malady and will know the best path forward. This is likely to be true, but you must still retain control of your overall care and treatment plan.

Whether you are reading this at the point where your physician is concerned about certain symptoms and wants to refer you to a specialist for additional diagnoses or you've moved beyond diagnosis and the next step is to begin treatment, know that you have choices. More than you might think.

Research—and Make—Your Choices of Physicians and Specialists

Most of us spend more time researching our next car than we do finding the person to whom we are entrusting our life. It is worth the time and effort to check ratings and reviews of doctors to make sure you will be comfortable with your clinicians. Just because someone is a highly esteemed professional does not make them the right person for you. As you build your care team, remember you do not need to accept the clinician to whom you have been initially referred.

You can find reliable information about clinicians at websites such as:

• Healthgrades.com
• Vitals.com

- WebMD.com
- Medicare Find and Compare Providers Near You: www .medicare.gov/care-compare (This site is really useful even if you aren't Medicare-eligible. It reports results for all Medicare patients at every clinician and facility that accepts Medicare.)
- On the web you can search for "doctor finder" websites in your state and community; they're often provided by healthcare organizations about their own physicians and by health insurance companies about the providers in their networks. There are also independent provider-finders like Medline Plus: https://medlineplus.gov/directories/.

Note that just because a clinician doesn't show up on one of these sites does *not* mean they aren't a good choice. Some of these sites depend on patient feedback, and there are many great physicians who don't receive five-star ratings from all their patients. But a physician with consistently low ratings is one to avoid.

You will also want to check with your insurance company's listing of in-network and out-of-network clinicians and facilities. A healthcare journey can be expensive, and you will want to strongly consider in-network clinicians, facilities, and treatments.

Questions to Ask Prospective Members of Your Care Team

When you meet potential members of your care team, ask them hard but respectful questions. Some examples:

- What is my diagnosis and prognosis?
- What is your experience with this specific disease?

- What should I, as your patient, expect? (This will help optimize your physical and mental responses to treatment.)
- What are your clinical outcomes treating this disease?
- If a loved one had this diagnosis, what would you recommend and where would you send them for treatment?
- Do you perform the procedures or does your staff?
- Who else will be on my care team, what will they do, and how experienced are they?
- What are the treatment alternatives we should consider?
- What can I do to increase my odds for success?
- Do you recommend a specific facility to use—and why do you recommend it?
- Should I get a second opinion?
- Where can I learn more?
- What support groups exist that I might join?
- Are there clinical trials I might participate in?

Involve Your Village

If it is right for you, share your thinking and research with your village. Bring one of them along when possible to interview clinicians you are considering.

One note about receiving advice from your village: You may know or meet someone who has the same condition you have or a similar one. Recommendations from friends and family—your village—are very helpful, but they should be balanced with other sources of information. Just because Uncle Bob loved his orthopedic surgeon does not mean that surgeon is the right one for you or the best expert to handle your specific condition.

Do Additional Research

Before committing to a specific team member and treatment direction, do research into treatment options. (Obviously, this works for something that is serious but not urgent. When care is needed immediately—a trauma surgery or treatment for a heart attack or stroke—you will have to do this research along the way.) In Step 1 we listed some of the many sources available to you for exploring your diagnosis, suggested treatments, and alternative and complementary options. You should continue to research different approaches as your treatment progresses—asking, for example, "Do I want an artificial or animal heart valve?" "What kind of surgical interventions are available?" "Are there immunotherapy treatments or clinical trials appropriate for my cancer?" "Which of the alternative medications is best for me?"

Firing a Member of Your Care Team

Once you have assembled a care team (and treatment may have started), you may decide you want someone off your care team. You may want to pick a substitute for one care team member, or you may want to put together a different care team altogether. Despite our best efforts, not all partnerships work out well.

Changing your care team may be necessary, but it should be approached carefully. Some healthcare organizations will be highly accommodating, some less so. In certain cases, changing your care team means having to go to a different facility. This is kind of a "nuclear option," because you may lose continuity of care or experience delays in care. Additionally, if you want to change one member of your care team, the remaining team members may become suspicious and overly cautious in their approach, fearing you will do the same with them.

So while changing care team members is a difficult and complicated matter, sometimes it is necessary and appropriate. Cris changed gastroenterologists when things weren't working well, for example. You can do it if you need to; just do it with as much grace as you can muster.

Step 3: Adding the Where to the Who

As we wrote earlier, you may want or need to begin by choosing your healthcare organization/facility and then selecting a care team within that organization. Or you might make those decisions in combination.

Whichever you do first, it's important to acknowledge that there are real differences between various clinics and hospitals and that your outcome can be strongly influenced by where you get care. It's an unfortunate truth that your zip code is often a better predictor of your

Dear Healthcare Colleagues,

This is a very personal book, arising from our experiences as patients and as leaders driving change in healthcare. And while most of the book is written for patients and families, we believe we gained insights by being in a hospital bed that cannot be gained by being around a hospital bed—and we want to share those with you too.

We know that healthcare is an imperfect yet ever-improving system full of well-intentioned institutions and people. That is what powers our hope that each patient will have a better healthcare experience tomorrow than he or she may have had yesterday. And that is why we want you to take a moment out of your demanding schedule to look at healthcare from the patient's point of view.

health than your genetic code. The hospital or clinic near you may be familiar, you may get your primary care there, and your village may say it's great, but you shouldn't necessarily limit yourself to what's in your area or what you're familiar with. If you are on a significant healthcare journey, you want to be treated in the place that's best for you, not necessarily the place that's nearest to you.

Also, as you talk with potential care team members you may find they are affiliated with specific hospitals. Ask the care team candidates if one location is better suited to address your medical needs than another.

So how do you, as the patient, decide where to get care? Do you even have that option given your geographic location, economic situation, family dynamics, and insurance coverage? And if your options are limited, how can you make sure you receive the most up-to-date, effective care possible?

Do Research and Ask Questions

Before you accept the facility of your clinician's choosing, do some research and ask your clinician a few questions.

- Why do you recommend this specific facility?
- How often do you practice there?
- Why is this facility preferred over the other options?
- How do the outcomes here compare to outcomes at other locations?

Some reliable online resources for finding and evaluating healthcare organizations include:

- *US News & World Report* rankings: https://health.usnews.com /best-hospitals
- Medicare Find and Compare Providers Near You: www .medicare.gov/care-compare/ (This site is really useful even if you aren't Medicare-eligible. It reports results for all Medicare patients at every clinician and facility that accepts Medicare.)
- WebMD: https://doctor.webmd.com/choice-awards
- MedlinePlus, a service of the National Library of Medicine: https://medlineplus.gov/directories/

Financial Considerations

Most hospitals will help you understand your costs before you make a commitment to be treated there. Some people might be afraid to commit to certain facilities for care because they think those places are too expensive. But remember, your cost of care is determined in large part by your insurance deductibles and co-pays. So in many cases the facility that might seem "too expensive" and the cheaper option may cost the same out of pocket, even if the rates they charge the insurance companies are different. Don't make the assumption that an excellent facility is out of reach financially until you've done some homework.

To Travel or Not to Travel?

Consider the convenience of location—but don't make that the only consideration. You may feel that a specific facility is best for you, but if it is three hours away, are you able and committed to making that commute as often as required? Are you willing to spend the resources needed on travel and perhaps on overnight accommodations? Can your village reach you and support you at a distance? Many times the answer to all those questions is yes. But be careful not to rush into such decisions until you have evaluated all the challenges, costs, and alternatives.

On the other hand, don't be afraid to travel. Insurance often covers medical procedures and surgeries done out of town or out of state. Research the best facilities in your region or nationally for your particular procedure. Then call the facilities and ask about your insurance coverage for all aspects of care there (room, anesthesia, surgery, doctor, other hospital charges—every possible aspect of care). Find out which specific doctors would provide treatment.

Finally, there has been interest in the last decade or so in "medical tourism"—where people travel to other countries for care that they believe is either better or cheaper. In the United States, the Medical Tourism Association (www.medicaltourismassociation.com) provides directories and other resources. As a disclaimer: Our hospitals, Mayo Clinic and Cleveland Clinic, are "destination medical centers," which welcome people from all states and many countries for treatment of serious and complex conditions. We believe in that model and know that travel allows many people to receive good care they can't get locally. We also know of people who have traveled to other countries for routine medical procedures—dental care, cosmetic procedures, orthopedic procedures, and so on—that can be provided at lower cost with quality equal to or better to that available in a US-based facility. And some people travel to other countries to receive emerging medical treatments not yet approved by the US Food and Drug Administration or the EU's European Medicines Agency. However, we also know that there are plenty of medically suspect, potentially low-quality, and dangerous treatment options outside the United States. Be careful.

Please research all healthcare facility choices with care and objective skepticism. When there is alignment between the data, science, your head, and your heart, you are ready to choose your care team.

A Breath of Fresh Air

For fifteen years Deb, now sixty-five, battled a relentless cough and chronic asthma. Finally she found relief working with a team of doctors who were empathetic and devoted the time and attention that was needed to provide her with what she describes as "miraculous relief."

> *Deb: I can't believe the difference in how I feel today. It brings me to tears to talk about it, because, after all those years, I was afraid I would never experience such an astounding difference in my quality of life.*
>
> *The short version of my story is that I developed a chronic cough fifteen years ago that my allergist diagnosed as asthma. But while he tried everything imaginable to treat it, nothing worked. Since he didn't know what else to do, he put me on a high daily dose of the steroid prednisone.*
>
> *Eventually he sent me for an MRI. It turned out I had nodules on my lungs, one of which was pretty good-sized. That meant I should see a pulmonologist. That doctor was so cold and said, "Well, we could do a biopsy to determine if the nodules are cancerous, but we might puncture your lung."*
>
> *I was scared. I might have cancer and the only way to be sure was to risk a punctured lung? I declined. So we did a PET scan instead, which indicated it wasn't cancer. But the pulmonologist offered no viable treatment options for my chronic cough and asthma. So I just kept taking massive doses of steroids.*

Then in the fall of 2022 I became feverish and exhausted. It persisted for three months. During those dark times, I was researching everything I could about my condition. I probably went overboard, but I truly believe you need to be your best advocate and go into every doctor's appointment well informed and with a written list of questions and concerns. Otherwise, too often you're just waiting for information from the doctor that never comes, and you walk out of the appointment clueless about what's going on.

My persistent chronic inflammation and low-grade fever led my primary care doctor to order another chest X-ray and then an MRI. Afterwards, the radiologist told me that I had metastatic lung disease caused by cancer elsewhere in the body that had moved into my lung.

I was devastated, but at the same time I thought of the scans from years ago, with the same nodules that were showing up today, more or less unchanged, so the cancer diagnosis didn't sit right.

I wanted a clear answer, so I went to an oncologist, who said he also did not think I had cancer, but he wanted a biopsy performed to definitively rule it out.

When the long ordeal of the biopsy was done, the radiologist looked at me and said, "Where is your husband?" I demanded to know what was going on. He told me that the needle got stuck in my lung and my lung had partially collapsed.

A thoracic surgeon was called immediately to take the tip of the needle out of my lung, and I was admitted to the hospital for an overnight stay. Three CT scans revealed no further collapse of my lung. However, the biopsy did not produce enough material to determine if the tissue was cancerous or not.

The oncologist then referred me to the pulmonology department in the same health system. I was exhausted and pessimistic, but they were amazing. Their goal was to get me off the 20 mg of prednisone that I had been taking daily for years. They even conjectured that it was the steroids that were aggravating my condition.

The pulmonologists there were my partners. In order for me to have access to new medications for severe asthma, they worked with me to get financial assistance to pay for the new medications. They also started me on a very gradual and safe step-down from steroids and prescribed a nebulizer—and they recommended nasal saline solutions to clear my nasal drainage. I was so excited when I began using these because it was the first time I could breathe clearly in decades! A month after I started the medications, I felt better than I had in years. Plus, I am down to 2.5 mg prednisone every other day and will soon be off the medication entirely.

The demeanor of the physicians means everything! My oncologist walked me out of the office into the waiting room like a father, with true concern about my physical and mental well-being. The physicians and the staff in the pulmonology department showed enormous compassion. It wasn't just that these doctors offered a more nuanced analysis of my condition; they offered me hope.

I know how much they care for me and how committed they are to improving my health. I truly believe that the mind and body work together and their compassionate care means everything to me.

It is important that a patient receives the respect they deserve and can trust the doctor to help them make the right decisions about their care. When I asked if we could adopt active surveillance and do follow-up CT scans to see if the nodules are growing (they haven't so far), the doctors agreed. We are in sync and I am feeling great.

My bonus: I am an inspirational speaker, and when I share difficult episodes in my life that, with prayer and God's help, I have received healing, I often tear up or flat-out cry. But when I do, I am confident that I will not have a debilitating coughing spell! It's a wonderful relief to have that absolute confidence.

Step 4: Understanding Your Care Path

Even after you have selected a clinician and a healthcare facility, there are still decisions to be made about how you will be diagnosed and treated. It's important that you understand options when they are available and work with your care team to decide what will happen next.

In Chapter 4 we wrote about things you should do to own your medical journey. Now that you have a care team and a care path is being defined, you should bring to the front all the things we emphasized in Chapter 4. Know that this is your journey. Gain resilience as you start down this path. Gain awareness. Integrate all that you can. This is when the journey really begins to unfold.

When the Steps Overlap

You may find that determining your care path overlaps or happens simultaneously with steps 1–3. This can happen, for example, when you are initially referred to a specialist who is an expert in your condition—something that might occur even before you have a full picture of your diagnosis. We recommend accepting the initial referral and meeting with this clinician unless you have strong reasons to want to be treated by someone else or at some other location than what your referring physician recommends. Then evaluate this clinician as a potential addition to your care team that will take you along your care path.

How Your Care Team Interacts on Your Care Path

Working closely with you on your care path will be the care team's lead physician. This clinician will interface with other specialists and oversee treatment choices and timing. For example, you may have an oncologist whom you see at each visit. That doctor coordinates with an oncological surgeon, anesthesiologist, rehabilitation physician, and so on. This is especially true in academic medical centers. In such facilities, you may also be treated by doctors in training (fellows or residents) who support your principal physician.

> *Ed's experience: When I had my prostatectomy, my primary physician did the actual surgery, but the opening and closing were done by a chief resident. There was yet another surgeon in residence who assisted my primary surgeon.*

> *Cris's experience: For me the chemotherapy choices seemed a given—they are standard protocol. For my second cancer I knew about proton beam radiation therapy and asked for it. Both of my surgeries were complex. For the second surgery I had six collaborating specialists. At Mayo, at least, the process includes a meeting of the patient with each surgeon.*
>
> *I found those meetings informative and reassuring. I was able to ask detailed questions and in some cases make choices that I would not have made without the meetings. For example, I knew that a fellow on the main surgical team would do much of the surgical procedure under supervision of the senior physician as a way of advancing his training. Initially, that made me a little*

apprehensive, but after meeting the senior physicians and their trainees I was perfectly OK with that. I knew the work would be coordinated and supervised by very skilled senior surgeons. I had also already expressed preferences to my surgeons about my desire for the most aggressive treatment needed to eliminate the cancer, but I didn't want an ostomy. My choices concerning chemo, surgical teams, and what I was willing to have done—or not done—defined my care path.

As much as possible, you want to:

- Know who is who on your care team, what they do, and at what stage they will be involved in your care.
- Know who is the most appropriate clinician for the questions you might have.
- Know who the human beings helping you are so that you can express gratitude to them.

Step 5: Solidifying Your Relationship with Your Care Team

You need to be able to create a dialogue with your care team so that you can ensure your care matches your preferences and choices. As wonderful and caring as clinicians are, they are responsible for many other patients. And they are pulled in competing directions, not only providing clinical input to dozens of patients but also fulfilling other healthcare ecosystem roles. All these activities take time and attention. While we patients want to believe the clinician's world revolves around us, that's not the case.

Finally, never forget that each clinician is a person like you. They have families to take care of and have their own personal and professional challenges. While they care immensely about you, no one will care as much about your success as you.

The Right Touch

1. Do not be shy about questioning your care team's decisions and choices. You can challenge opinions respectfully.
2. Practice excellent people and relationship skills.
3. Practice kindness and gratitude even in the midst of pain. It is human nature that the better you treat someone, the better they will treat you.

Tips for Interacting with Your Care Team Members

- Write down questions beforehand and share them with the principal members of your care team. Consider bringing two copies of your questions to office visits—one for you and one to give to your physician. We have also written questions for ourselves on our mobile phones and used our notes to remember what to ask. In addition, consider sharing the questions with one or more people in your village. They may help you shape the questions, add their own, and gain greater understanding of what you are facing physically and emotionally.
- Listen before asking questions or talking. Take notes or have them taken for you.
- Don't think that the clinicians know everything. They need input from you about your condition, how you are feeling, your

worries, what you need more information about. They may
have overlooked something, or you may have a symptom or
concern that you've downplayed or forgotten to mention. Don't
clam up!

- If you've received advice or have found information online and
want to know more about it or want it to be considered for
your care, share it. Clinicians want you to be empowered. But
also understand that physicians hear often from patients who
have been "diagnosed and treated by Dr. Google." They are
right to be skeptical about "the new hidden treatment that Big
Pharma doesn't want revealed" that you read about on social
media. Remember that your care team is the team you want to
be on. Don't fight the team; help the team.

- At the end of an appointment, be sure to summarize what
you've been told and get confirmation that you understand
it correctly. Take your time. Make sure you know about the
frequency of medications, time between your next visits,
physical therapy, exercise recommendations, and so on. This
way, when you leave, everyone is in agreement on next steps.

- If needed, use or ask for visual aids such as graphs, pain scales,
or time charts to communicate with your physician—anything
that will help clarify your questions or concerns. If you have
documented something important—you've charted your
changing levels of pain on a graph, for example—you can leave
this information with the clinician so they can review later
and, as appropriate, add to your medical records.

- Talk to nurses. While we all want to speak directly with the
physician every time, a nurse can be the most knowledgeable

and reachable person on your care team. They often have more time available than doctors do, and they often serve as a trusted partner to the doctor and can give you expert advice. Cris credits the nurses in oncology for helping him understand and manage anti-nausea medications and the nurse-partner to his surgeon for telling him how to manage symptoms after surgery. Consider nurses as advocates of your care.

Your Job as a Care Team Member

Once you have agreed to a treatment plan, it is your role to follow your treatment plan with authenticity, transparency, and accountability. You may be surprised to learn that less than half of all medications prescribed are ever picked up, and fewer are actually taken as directed. Patients tend to not follow through on clinicians' directions related to physical therapy or behavioral changes. You need to follow the treatment plan to be a good partner in your care plan.

Remember, you are the leader of this care team. You need to lead by example. You would be dismayed to find out your clinician did not carry out the duties they had agreed to. You would be upset if a member of the village dropped the ball on something critical to your well-being. In the same way, you want to be a strong leader, a trustworthy partner. So be a leader, but follow the advice and treatment plan you helped develop and agreed to. After all, it is your health that is at stake.

Step 6: Introducing Village Members to Your Care Team

When possible, bring a key member of your village with you when meeting a care team member. As we've said, when you are the patient it's tough to hear and remember everything that is being thrown at you.

Especially when you are receiving a diagnosis or important information about the course of your treatment, shock can set in. You may not retain all the information shared with you. Having someone there to ask questions for you, write down what the clinician says, and recap the experience with you afterward is helpful. We both took notes, but we found we didn't recall all the intent of the words when we reviewed them later.

Share information between your care team and your village. For example, we shared the names of our principal physicians with the key members of our village. We shared with our village when we were going to be hospitalized and where we were in the hospital. We also shared information about our village with our care team. They wanted to know about our support structure—who was going to pick us up, who would be at home to take care of us when we were discharged. They wanted to know who our visitors were when we were hospitalized and whom to contact in the event further collaboration was required. We found that it gave our care team confidence in the success of our journey when they saw a support mechanism in action.

Step 7: Remember to Recognize Team Members for Their Contributions to Your Welfare

As you build a close and effective relationship with your care team, you may discover that you want them to know how much you appreciate their efforts on your behalf. If you want to take that extra step, note down (on paper or your cell phone) the members of your care team and keep it handy. Keep this list fresh as members of your care team change. Share the updated list whenever you make a change so that everyone has the most current information.

We considered everyone we encountered during our care as a part of our care team. Ed counted eighty-eight people in total; Cris counted over a hundred. That included doctors and nurses, of course, but also radiology techs, phlebotomists, radiation oncology techs, medical assistants, housekeeping staff, receptionists, and transport staff. They all had an important role to play in our treatment and recovery, even if it was just a smile or a random act of kindness. It all mattered. We wrote down their names so we would never forget them. You can decide how far you want to go with this.

When Cris was hospitalized, he took a cell phone picture of a big bulletin board that displayed photos of everyone who worked on that particular floor. Whenever he was moved to a new floor, he took a new picture. It helped him remember names and address people by their names when he encountered them. Ed added the names and roles of all the clinicians he encountered on his phone calendar and then combined the lists at the end of his journey.

Action Steps: Putting Together Your Care Team

1. Identify your care team. Write out their names and specific roles. You may want to name your care team; it could be as simple as Care Team Ross or Care Team Marx, or it could be something more creative or inspiring, like Cancer Killers or Valiant Protectors of the Heart. (Guess which one of us came up with those last two names.)

2. Ensure that your care team record includes the physical locations and detailed contact info for where you will

receive treatment. These may include a clinical office, a hospital, a physical therapy center, and so on. Collect phone numbers for the specific areas where you get care, so that when you want to change an appointment, for example, you won't get routed to a general appointment line, where you might get the runaround.

3. In Chapter 4 we recommended that you start a record of your intentions for your healthcare journey. Initially, this is just for you—to clarify how you are feeling and where you are hoping to end up. With that as a foundation, we suggest you add to this by documenting your intentions for your care team: a short description of your health challenge, your intentions, and your ideal outcomes.

4. If it's right for you, share all or some of your written hopes or expectations with your care team. This will help keep everyone on the same page and contribute to continued engagement. All members will have a shared understanding of your situation and your preferred outcome. This shared knowledge will help your care team rally around you. Here are some examples of what we shared with our care teams:

   - Please give me the most aggressive treatments that I can endure to maximize my chances for survival.
   - In surgery, I am willing to accept a higher risk of recurrence of cancer if I can avoid permanent damage to my body.
   - Please challenge me in rehabilitation so I can regain my health and vitality.

———

Congratulations! At this point, hopefully, you are clear about your intentions, you have assembled a village to support you, and you have selected a care team and are aligned with them. Now you are more than ready to make sure your treatment journey is as positive, effective, and reassuring as possible.

One more thing: The fact you have read this far says a lot about you. As we write, we are thinking about you. We have never met, but now we are bonded to one another. Keep fighting.

Seven

Your Best-Care Checklists

*Daily guides to checking in with
yourself and interacting with your teams*

Congratulations on getting this far. We understand many of the emotions you must be going through right now as you navigate this health journey. (Or if you are a caregiver reading this book for the benefit of someone else, the emotions you are encountering plus the burdens you are taking on.) Taking the time to read a book in the midst of this requires concentration, so we wanted to make this as easy as possible by summarizing the main points from the last three chapters. Being your own advocate and owning your own journey, establishing your village, and building your care team are undoubtedly the most critical to ensuring your optimal experience.

However, it is important to realize that making sure you have the best experience and receive the medical care that's optimal for you is an ongoing process—one you need to keep tabs on as you progress through diagnosis, acute or ongoing treatment, and recovery. So we've provided some checklists to help you keep tabs on all these stages.

- **Yourself Checklist.** How are you doing? How have you advocated for yourself? How can you make yourself feel better?
- **Your Diagnosis and Your Questions Checklist.** Tracking the often-overwhelming info you are given surrounding your diagnosis.
- **Your Village Checklist.** What else do you need? What do you need less of? Who's sticking to their tasks; who's not? Who needs to be added, reinforced, or even ignored or politely removed?
- **Your Care Team Checklist.** A list of all the clinicians you have interacted with or are slated to work with and their contact information.
- **Your What You Want to Do When You Don't Have to Think About All This Checklist.**

Yourself Checklist

The function of this checklist is to help you keep track of how you are doing, how you have advocated for yourself, and how you can make yourself feel better. This needs to be filled in frequently, probably weekly—you'll be surprised how your mood, attitude, and behaviors change during the course of this journey.

Here are the main points to help make sure you are doing as well as possible through this journey.

1. You own this journey. It's sometimes hard to remember this, but you are the one driving the car (loaded with people) that takes you through this experience. You may forget it in the moment because of your own emotions,

but this is about *you*. Self-advocacy is not just OK, it is critical. In some cases you may need help advocating for yourself. Sometimes a village member—a spouse or partner—may step up as your fiercest advocate. But even if you are unable to advocate for yourself, it is *you* who appoints a member of your village to serve as your principal advocate.

2. Attend to building your resilience. Anyone can do it! Eat well, take time for rest, cultivate and gain strength from relationships, try journaling, go for walks, pray, laugh, do things you enjoy—whatever you need. While building resilience and maintaining a positive attitude (one of the results of resilience) may or may not lead directly to positive medical outcomes, it will vastly improve your quality of life.

∽

YOURSELF CHECKLIST

› How would you describe how you are feeling about your diagnosis and/or treatment? Three to five words is fine; sentences are OK. _____

_____

_____

› How are you feeling about your expected or hoped-for outcome? Three to five words is fine; sentences are OK. _____

_____

_____

› Write a brief explanation of what you don't understand about your diag-nosis. Do you feel you lack information? Are your clinicians not good at explaining things? Could it be that your confusion is because you don't want to hear things or your emotions keep you from hearing fully or clearly? All of the above? _____

_____

_____

› Write what you imagine to be your "best self" as you go through treatment. As we described in Chapter 4, we believe that no particular stance toward treatment is objectively best. Rather, what is best for you? Think how you can be that person. Write down your ideas.

_____

_____

› What activities can you do regularly that decrease your stress and build your resilience? These may include meditation, exercise, conversations with friends, reading, a hobby, talking to your plants—anything that works for you! It's important to commit to self-care.

_____

_____

_____

› Assess how well you have interacted with your village members (no matter if there are many or few participants, or whether they are local or far afield). Creating support is essential for optimal quality of life.

_____

_____

_____

› Evaluate how well you are following your doctors' recommendations for medication adherence, diet, sleep, physical activities, lifestyle, or behavior changes and so on. What can you do to improve your compliance? How can you ask your village for help? How can you ask your doctor for help?

_____

_____

_____

Your Diagnosis and Questions Checklist

Keeping track of your diagnosis and the often-overwhelming information you receive can be challenging. Remembering the order of various steps and procedures (which may have weird acronyms or names that seem unpronounceable) isn't something you can just keep in your head—you need to write it all down or have someone from your village who goes to the appointments with you write it down.

YOUR DIAGNOSIS AND QUESTIONS CHECKLIST

› I have been diagnosed with _____

_____

_____

› If it is designated with a stage or degree of severity, that is _____

› My expected treatment duration is _____
my treatment plan includes _____
and my outcome is expected to be _____

› The treatment choices are (check those that apply):

☐ Vigilant watching

☐ Nonsurgical intervention

☐ Surgery

☐ Medication, chemotherapy, radiation therapy, etc.

☐ Implantation of a device

☐ Other form of treatment

› What are my choices? What are the risks and benefits of my choices?

_____

_____

_____

_____

_____

If you don't know the answers to any of the questions above, schedule a phone conversation / have a virtual visit / get an in-office appointment with your doctor(s) / send a message to your care team to communicate specifically about these issues. Get at least one village member involved in this discussion too so they can help interpret things, ask questions for you, or remember things for you.

› The choice(s) I want to make are:

_____

_____

_____

_____

_____

Your Village Checklist

Your village consists of family and friends who care about you and are willing to commit to helping you—and, as needed, help your family or household—as you go through your journey. It may be a large number of individuals or a handful of people closest to you. Key trusted village members should provide another set of ears and eyes for you during clinical visits and be present for you emotionally and physically as you receive information, get treatment, or have discussions with your clinicians. Other key village members can help with day-to-day tasks. That could be running errands, doing tasks for you, volunteering to bring food, taking your kids to soccer practice—whatever you might need.

Your checklist should help you be honest about who's sticking with you and who's not; who else you need to participate in your village; how you can be better at asking for help; and (in some cases) who should be ignored or politely dismissed from the village.

It's important to remember that people who are highly involved either directly or emotionally with your journey are going through a journey too. Some will do better than others; some will find they don't have the time, or they will get too involved and bring distracting emotions or drama to your journey. You want to let some people move off your team, reinforce those who are staying, and add new members if needed and/or possible.

Caregivers need your appreciation—and they need you to recognize that your journey can be an emotional roller coaster for them too. You need to work together. Hopefully this checklist will help you put together the best support team possible and care for them as they care for you.

YOUR VILLAGE CHECKLIST

› What are your greatest needs for help right now? List all of them. (For those of you who struggle to ask for help, use this as an opportunity to stretch a little!) _____

_____

_____

_____

› Which members of your village have been most effective at meeting the needs you just listed? It might be that your sister is best at going to medical appointments and understanding medical needs, and your neighbor helps best by taking care of your dogs. Think of this as a list of what you need and who is showing up best to help you. _____

_____

_____

_____

› Who wants to help but hasn't been able to do so? If possible, find a job for them to do even if it isn't your highest priority. It will make both of you feel better. List the possible helpers and what you want them to do.

_____

_____

_____

_____

Reach out and communicate how they might help you on your journey (for example, grocery shop once a week; set up a regular phone call with you; help you do your laundry; walk the dog; call you up with a joke every day; go with you to a doctor's appointment). You'll be surprised how grateful people can be for the chance to do something that is genuinely helpful to you. They might be overwhelmed by your situation and appreciate a concrete request for help.

› An especially hard question: Who on the team is not helpful or is getting in the way? Whom would you like to ease off the team or have do less? List them and specify either a potential alternative assignment for them or a way to say, "No, thank you."

_____

_____

This can be delicate, but if there is someone who is driving you nuts with their helicopter worrying, unhelpful advice, or prying manner, you are allowed to remove that stress from your daily life. Talk to a family or village member you are particularly close with and ask for help deflecting the person, or give the bothersome village member "assignments" that don't involve seeing you. And you are always welcome to say, "Thank you for suggesting that you come over, but I am not up for it today."

Your Care Team Checklist

The care team is made up of everyone who provides medical and supportive care as well as medical institutions such as hospitals and clinics. They work with you to create a treatment plan and define the path and milestones for care. The rapport you establish with your care team is vital to your experience. It is OK for you to assert yourself and ensure your needs are being met, but you also need to establish strong relationships and good communication with all key people involved in your care. It's also important to adopt a stance of gratitude and grace. These people are in your life in an intimate way, even if only for a brief period of time. We found that our best selves through our journeys often lived in grace and gratitude.

So, make a list (see below) of all the doctors and other healthcare professionals, such as physical therapists and nutritionists, you have interacted with or are slated to work with and their contact information—as well as notes to yourself and your village about how they behave, what you like or don't like about them, and concerns you may have. Also, it is helpful to add support staff you interact with.

〜

YOUR CARE TEAM CHECKLIST

› Doctors I have seen, their specialty, and their role in my diagnosis and care:

1. _____   _____   _____
          (name)   (contact info)   (specialty)

   _____   _____
      (role in my diagnosis)   (role in my care)

   Member of support staff (PA, nurse, front desk, etc.) _____

   Comments: _____

2. _____   _____   _____
          (name)   (contact info)   (specialty)

   _____   _____
      (role in my diagnosis)   (role in my care)

   Member of support staff (PA, nurse, front desk, etc.) _____

   Comments: _____

3. _____   _____   _____
          (name)   (contact info)   (specialty)

   _____   _____
      (role in my diagnosis)   (role in my care)

   Member of support staff (PA, nurse, front desk, etc.) _____

   Comments: _____

Lather, rinse, repeat!

Your What You Want to Do When You Don't Have to Think About All This Checklist

Let yourself look forward to post-treatment days and interactions with the world. Set some pleasurable goals for down the road—activities, places to go, people to see, books to read, meals to cook, vegetables to plant. Cris made plans to re-landscape his backyard. Ed challenged Cris to climb a mountain when his leg has fully recovered its strength (that's in sight!). We know someone who put her wishes on little pieces of paper and placed them under her pillow at night so she could dream of better days.

You may ask, "What if my journey has an uncertain or limited future?" If so, we're sorry. Neither of us received a diagnosis of a late-stage or terminal illness, but we did confront the possibilities that our illness could end our lives. Out-of-date—but still scary—survival tables say Cris has a 10 percent chance of being alive five years after ending his second journey through cancer. He intends to beat the odds.

In significant ways our treatments have impaired us. If you have a limited or uncertain future, remember that you can still live with purpose. For us, that meant seeking to "find the gifts" of our illnesses and living with joy and intention.

There are terrific resources, often within the disease-specific websites or support groups we listed in Chapter 6, to help you if your diagnosis is potentially dire. The National Institute on Aging has great information about palliative and hospice care (www.nia.nih.gov/health/what-are -palliative-care-and-hospice-care) regardless of your age. These sources can help guide you in important ways. Godspeed.

You may choose or not choose to use this checklist depending how formal you are with these kinds of things. There is no right or wrong way. This checklist is just meant to stimulate some ideas and thoughts.

You may choose to add some other items or just use a handful. Whatever works for you. Here are some questions you may want to ask yourself, and ideas for helping you as you transition into this next phase.

WHAT YOU WANT TO DO WHEN YOU DON'T HAVE TO THINK ABOUT ALL THIS CHECKLIST

In the First 30 Days

› Give yourself permission to grieve.

› Give yourself permission to feel joy.

› What are your plans to restore yourself to your new normal? _____

_____

› How do you want to celebrate your journey, if at all?_____

_____

In the First 90 Days

› Are there relationships (maybe inside your Village) that you want to focus on?

_____

› Would you like to do or get something to indulge yourself after your difficult journey? _____

› Do you need to show gratitude to anyone? If yes, how? _____

_____

› What promises did you make to yourself and others that you should take
action on? _____

› Are there relationships that need attention, repair, restoration? _____

_____

› Getting away — Is there someplace you thought you might go when all this
was over? _____

› Was there someone you wanted to go with you? _____

_____

In the First Year

› Do you want to celebrate a One-Year Anniversary? If yes, how and with
whom? _____

› Do you need to check in on any promises previously made to yourself or
others? _____

If Time Is Limited

› If your journey is uncertain or your future limited, what is important to do in
your remaining time? _____

› Who are you at this phase of your journey? _____

Putting the Pieces Together

Whatever works for you on this health journey is the right approach. These chapters contain some of our best advice, garnered from hard-won experience, as well as valuable input from our colleagues in the field of healthcare. We hope they help you find resilience and even moments of joy and grace through the toughest times. We'd be honored to join your village. Consider us a hand you can hold through your healthcare journey. Now on to "the System" and its pitfalls.

Eight

The Mysteries of Medical Care in America

*Unraveling your biggest questions
about how healthcare is delivered*

When we set out to write this book, we wanted to bring two things: an honest account of our firsthand experiences as patients and insight from our experience as healthcare executives. This chapter is a blend of those two goals. It offers a look at what we and other patients experience that is bewildering and maddening about the healthcare system and what we two, as healthcare insiders, understand are the reasons that certain obstacles exist to optimal and easy-to-get care. Some of those reasons make sense; some are unacceptable and need to be changed.

We have divided the chapter into two sections: one dealing with what we consider to be big issues and one dealing with things we consider annoying. We want to provide some inside perspectives on big issues because your ability to navigate around and through them may have an effect on the quality of your care. And we want to provide some information about annoying things because your ability to avoid or cope with them may make your journey more tolerable.

Most people who work in healthcare know we can do better. *So why don't you?* you might ask. The short version is that we work at it every day, and we can give examples of how things are becoming better: new therapies that have made terminal illnesses into chronic diseases, technologies that make accessing healthcare more convenient, improvements in quality care in smaller facilities and rural areas (with a long way still to go) and so on. But plenty of things are still broken.

Five Big Issues: What They Are and How to Handle Them

1. Delayed Effective Treatment

One 2022 study showed the average wait time in the United States to get a primary care appointment was eighteen days. In some areas, patients waited an average of thirty-two days. And the latest report on wait times for specialists, from Merritt Hawkins, an offshoot of the physician search firm AMN Healthcare, says wait times are up 8 percent since 2017; it now takes around twenty-six days for a new patient to get in to see a medical specialist. In some places it is even worse than that. They found that in Portland, Oregon, some patients wait eighty-four days to see a dermatologist. To see a cardiologist, the average wait time was more than twenty-six days, up from around twenty-one days in 2017. And these delays are in metropolitan areas—rural areas are even harder hit.

If you are reading this outside the United States, you know that delays may be worse where you live. In Canada, the Fraser Institute reports that the wait time from a referral by a general practitioner to a consultation with a specialist averaged 11.1 weeks in 2021, and time from referral to a specialist to treatment averaged 14.5 weeks. In the United Kingdom, the *Guardian* reports that in 2022, nearly 40 percent of NHS hospital departments have average treatment waiting times above 18 weeks—with average waits at some well over 30 weeks. The Organisation for Economic Co-operation and Development, a consortium of generally well-off countries, measured wait times in many countries in 2010, 2013, and 2016 and found that the United States was on par with the Netherlands, Germany, and Switzerland and that wait times are longer in Canada, Norway, Sweden, New Zealand, the United Kingdom, Australia, and France.

Why Does It Take So Long to Get an Appointment?
First, there is a shortage of doctors nationwide (and worldwide)—especially primary care doctors. The US government estimates the country needs 15,000 more primary care physicians (PCPs) just to meet current shortfalls, and the association of American Medical Colleges estimates there could be a shortfall of somewhere between 17,000 and 48,000 PCPs by 2034.

Specialists are hard to see for other reasons—an ever-increasing number of older people needing ever more specialized care, for one thing, and the expansion of insurance coverage (a great thing) putting more people in line for specialized care, for another.

What you can do to reduce your wait time:

- At a PCP or specialist's office, ask about adding your name to a cancellation list so you can get an earlier appointment if one becomes available.
- See if a second location for the same healthcare organization, PCP, or specialist's practice might see you sooner.

- Get your PCP to contact a specialist you want to see directly on your behalf. There's usually built-in flexibility even in a "full schedule" that doctor-to-doctor conversations may open up. You might even ask your PCP to consult with a specialist via a video call to see if the PCP can learn how to help take care of your immediate problem(s) or concerns.
- Ask if the hospital, healthcare system, or practice has a service dedicated to finding how to escalate an appointment request. Many large organizations do.

Transitioning to Better Care: Amelia's Story

People who are trans or gender-nonconforming often face enormous challenges when dealing with the healthcare system. It can be difficult to get an appointment with any doctor in some locations, and even harder finding a doctor with knowledge of the health issues related to transitioning.

> *Amelia: I had to get a new primary care doctor when I was transitioning, and it took me about three years to find someone. I knew a mental health therapist who was tuned in to transgender identities, and she had a recommendation—but the doctor was twenty-five miles away and I don't have a car, so I couldn't do that. And then there were other obstacles, like insurance and being able to register as transgender.*
>
> *When I did finally identify a doctor, it took six months to get an appointment. There are great clinics in NYC for people transitioning, with no openings. And even once you get set up with initial medical care it can be rough going. Mount Sinai has a clinic for transgender medicine, but it took a long time to get an appointment and eighteen months to get*

surgical care. The upside to that difficult process? They have a great team and provide excellent care.

I think it's important for everyone who is somewhere without any resources to know that telehealth is a good alternative. It is one of the main reasons trans people can access healthcare—and you can go anywhere to get your labs.

Because of the growing attack on trans healthcare, you have to find your community. My message is you have to find and/or build a trans community. That's who is going to help you the most and support you and provide references. Find other trans people and sit down with them over coffee and chat with them about how they have been able to access healthcare.

Also know that you may experience all kinds of rejection—subtle and overt—from healthcare providers. I went to an emergency care clinic once and they chased me out of there. . . . Even when my primary referred me to an endocrinologist and they worked together and they could refer me to a mental health person, I still had to interview the therapists; it was hit-and-miss. But keep at it, talk to lots of people about what they are doing, and don't settle.

Why Can't I Go to the Hospital or Clinic I Want?

You may have gotten advice from your primary care physician, checked in with your village, searched the internet and read books, and now you know exactly where you want to be treated and by whom. One problem: your health insurance policy doesn't recognize that provider as "in-network." That means that you will have to pay a much higher co-pay until you reach your out-of-pocket limit, or perhaps your deductible will be higher for out-of-network care.

Insurance companies almost always negotiate with hospitals and clinics about whether they will be in-network or not. In a large metropolitan area or an area with lots of competition among healthcare systems, organizations have less leverage in negotiations and may have to either accept lower reimbursement levels or agree not to be part of that insurer's network.

Furthermore, insurance companies, trying to reduce the cost of premiums to employers and to you, sometimes have "narrow networks"—they include only a few providers who are willing to accept the lowest possible reimbursement rates.

You or a loved one may have had the experience of purchasing a health insurance policy with a really low premium, which seemed good at the time, only to find that when you face a difficult diagnosis you can't get care at the place you want to be treated because it is out-of-network and the resulting co-pays or deductible is too expensive.

If you have Medicare, generally it will pay any hospital or clinic in good standing that agrees to be paid at Medicare reimbursement levels and under their other conditions.

What you can do to get treatment with the doctor or hospital you want:

- If your doctor or clinic is out-of-network and there is an available in-network provider, your options to get care paid for may be limited. However, in some circumstances the in-network providers may not be accepting new patients, or the distance to an in-network provider may be excessive. We know of situations like these where an insurance company agreed to reimburse the provider as in-network. Caution: if the network in your area changes and an in-network provider becomes available, you may have a difficult financial choice—whether to continue with the provider who is seeing you but pay out-of-network rates, or switch to the in-network provider.

- Do the math. Depending on the severity of your health situation, you may find that your deductible is a financial burden—and then what you have to pay once coverage kicks in is not trivial. For example, you may have a $3,000 to $10,000 yearly deductible, and once that is reached your co-pay is 50 percent for out-of-network providers and 10 percent for in-network providers. It is helpful to know up front what kind of bills you may be looking at. Contact your insurance company and ask them to work with you to understand what you are likely to pay for the treatments and care that is ahead of you. Also ask about possible lifetime limits on coverage and/or restrictions on which care providers you can use and what treatments are covered—or not.

Why Am I Required to Undergo Tests That Seem Duplicative or Not Very Helpful?

One example of this is imaging. You may be asked to have an X-ray before getting a CT scan or MRI. An X-ray is the least expensive and quickest way to obtain an image, and before ordering an expensive CT or MRI exam, a physician may want to use a fast and simple X-ray to rule out obvious problems. In general, physicians err on the side of conservative or cautious approaches to care (for example, physical therapy as a first line for treatment of a painful shoulder, rather than more intrusive and expensive treatments like surgery).

You also might be told to get a duplicate image if you had a CT scan at one hospital but are now receiving treatment at another facility. This happens for several reasons. Not all imaging studies are exactly the same, and your body can be placed in different positions. Your first scan may not have been done using a contrast medium, an injected compound that provides a clearer view of what's going on inside you. And different scans may have different levels of resolution, changing the quality of the image.

You also may have repeated blood and urine tests. That can happen if the first test(s) looked at the particular things that now need to be measured regularly. Blood and urine are usually kept for a few days so more tests can be run on the original samples, but after that, fresh blood and urine samples are needed. Also, your body chemistry can change over the course of a few days. If you're being diagnosed for something significant, your physician will want to have the most timely information. You might not like to get poked or to pee in a cup, but the benefits are very significant.

What you can do to avoid unnecessary or duplicative tests:

- If you've already had imaging studies, make sure your new physician knows about them. Sometimes tests are ordered somewhat routinely, so let the new doctor know what you've already had done.
- Bring your old images with you. This is one of these maddening things that we (like us two guys in healthcare tech) should have fixed by now. Most data moves pretty well from health system to health system, but imaging studies are complex, large data files that can make transfers difficult. These

are stupid, solvable technical details, so why haven't we made it easy to have them taken in one place and read in another? Believe us, we're working on it!

- If you are changing health systems, you may need to ask the old hospital to put your images on a DVD (so 1990s, right?) or ask them to digitally transfer them to the new hospital. Or you can ask the new hospital to request the files from the old hospital. Honestly, it can be a hassle to get these images moved, and sometimes there can be a bias that they don't do them as well "over there." Ask anyway. Be persistent.

- If you had a blood or urine test in the last few days at a particular hospital, all departments and physicians should have access to the results. If some caregiver isn't aware of it, ask why your test from a few days ago needs to be repeated. Even if the test was done in a different lab, if it was done within the last few days ask to have the old sample retested for whatever new thing your doctor wants to check.

Why Can't I Get the Specific Treatment That I Know I Need?

This perplexing dilemma comes in at least two flavors. One, you've learned about a treatment and you're convinced it's right for you, but your care team disagrees. Two, you and your doctor prefer a course of treatment, but the insurance company won't pay for it.

You and your care team disagree. If you want your care team to provide a treatment and they decline to offer it, first seek to understand why. It's all part of owning your own health journey. If in the end you don't agree because your care team thinks a treatment is inappropriate or too risky or not within their area of expertise, consider getting a new care team (see Chapter 6). On the other hand, consider the possibility that the miracle cure that you learned about on social media or that your friend's cousin swears by really isn't medically advised and your care team is on solid science-based ground.

Your hospital disagrees with you and your care team. In some rare circumstances for a rare condition, a physician may want to try a particular treatment but hospital management won't support it. In those circumstances ask yourself why your doctor is in favor of something that their peers and managers don't agree to. It could be that you have the right doctor but the wrong hospital. If so, maybe you and your doctor have some options. But if there is such a difference between what your doctor wants to try and what the facility will allow, it's most likely because the consensus of opinion is that the treatment is not medically indicated for you. A hospital saying no is a flashing yellow light or even a red one.

Your insurance company is stalling or saying no. If your insurance company won't pay for a recommended treatment that you and your doctor are in favor of, it might be because the treatment is unusual, unknown, or expensive. It can also be because they require "prior authorization" before they will pay for it, and getting that can be time-consuming and tricky.

In either case, if you and your care team feel that a treatment is right for you but it is not covered by insurance or accessing it is difficult because of a requirement for prior authorization, push your doctor, clinic, and/or hospital to do the extra administrative work to get what you and the team think is right for you. Sometimes it comes down to convincing an administrative person to take on a difficult assignment.

The high cost of care. As we mentioned, sometimes insurance denies coverage simply because the treatment is too expensive. This can happen whether your medical care is paid for by the government (through Medicare, Medicaid, the Veterans Administration, or the military), by private insurance companies, or out of your pocket.

Everyone knows that healthcare in the United States costs more than it should. Why does this happen? People have different opinions about why healthcare costs so much: our demographics; too many fancy hospital buildings and too few patients; the huge cost of research and development of new therapies; health insurance company profits; Big Pharma's greediness; hospital executives like us (Cris and Ed) being paid too much; the FDA blocks cheap miracle treatments; clinician salaries; and on and on.

As healthcare executives, we think healthcare is expensive for lots of reasons, some good and some bad, but we work every day to help deliver better treatments at lower cost. As patients, we won't say that money is no object, but we sought the best available care where we could, and you should too. Cris knew that proton beam radiation therapy might cost more than standard radiation therapy, but he also knew how much damage he had incurred from standard treatment and so advocated for himself to get proton beam treatment. (It turns out Mayo Clinic generally charges the same for equivalent courses of either treatment.)

If you are required to get a prior authorization for a treatment or medication and it is denied—that is, you went the right route, but even then it didn't work—you can appeal. There are a couple of ways you (or your doctor) can do this. The documentation that accompanies the denial will provide contact information for both routes.

- **Peer-to-peer review.** The insurance company's staff medical professional can speak to your doctor and decide if the denial should be overridden.
- **Appeal.** An appeal requires that you or your doctor write a letter to the insurance company explaining why the procedure (or product, or medication) is essential for treatment.

Is it worth appealing? A study by the Kaiser Family Foundation of Medicare Advantage plans found that 35 million prior authorization requests were made in 2021, and that 2 million (6 percent) were fully or partially denied by Medicare. Of the 2 million that were denied, only 11 percent were appealed. But of those that were appealed, 82 percent were overturned. Results for private insurers will vary. But the bottom line is that it's worth it for your doctor to seek prior authorization and for you to appeal denials.

Does the prior authorization process make sense if 82 percent of appeals are successful? Most healthcare providers want to fix that process or make it go away because it is an administrative hassle and can delay care. We also understand that governments and insurance companies seeking to control how much healthcare costs have limited tools: deciding who is in-network, negotiating what a doctor or hospital will be paid for a certain service, and controlling access to the highest-cost treatments except where medical need demands it. We're not trying to judge whether it's right or not, but that is how things work today.

2. Unexpected Expenses for Doctors and Treatments

Effective January 1, 2022, the No Surprises Act protects you from surprise billing if you have a group health plan or group or individual health insurance coverage. It prohibits what is called out-of-network cost-sharing, also known as out-of-network co-insurance or co-payments, for all emergency and some nonemergency services. It also says you cannot receive surprise bills for emergency services from an out-of-network provider or facility without prior authorization—and it bans out-of-network charges and balance bills for supplemental care, like radiology or anesthesiology, by out-of-network providers who work at an in-network facility.

The No Surprises Act also requires some healthcare institutions and providers to let you know what local, state, and national provisions exist to protect you from surprise billing and how to lodge a complaint if you need to.

In addition, the law looks out for people who don't have health insurance and those who pay for care without using health insurance. The institution providing care is required to give you a good-faith estimate of costs before you get care (but make sure you ask for it). If the final cost is more than $400 above the good-faith estimate, you can dispute the charges.

People who are on Medicare or Medicaid or who use Indian Health Services, Veterans Affairs Health Care, or TRICARE are also protected from surprise billing.

When a surprise bill happens because some out-of-network service or provider is added to your care, you usually only need to pay your normal in-network costs (like co-insurance, co-payments, and amounts paid toward deductibles). It's your health insurance plan and the provider who have to duke it out—nothing to do with you!

What Do I Do If I End Up with an Unexpected Bill for Medical Care?
Because this can still happen despite the No Surprises Act, there are
steps you can take to resolve the issue.

- To learn more about the No Surprises Act, check out www
  .cms.gov/nosurprises. To lodge a complaint if the act is not
  being followed, contact the Centers for Medicare and Medicaid
  Services No Surprises Help Desk at 1-800-985-3059 from
  8 a.m. to 8 p.m. EST, 7 days a week. You can also go online to
  file a complaint at www.CMS.gov/nosurprises/consumers
  /complaints-about-medical-billing.
- The Consumer Assistance Program at the Centers for Medicare
  and Medicaid Services (www.CMS.gov/cciio/resources
  /consumer-assistance-grants) can also help with problems,
  questions, and complaints. And check out the Centers for
  Medicare and Medicaid Services online at No Surprises Act |
  CMS (www.cms.gov/nosurprises).

*What Can I Do to Reduce Medical Costs If I Am Underinsured or
Don't Have Any Insurance?*
It can be horrifying to contemplate what a visit to the ER or a surgery
could cost someone without sufficient insurance or without any insurance
at all. Fortunately, there are ways to reduce the financial burden and
even eliminate it if you are under- or uninsured.

- The Affordable Care Act (ACA) requires nonprofit hospitals to
  have a written financial assistance policy (FAP) and a written
  emergency medical care policy—and they have to let you know

about them. In addition, when you are discharged the hospital must offer you a sheet that outlines steps to take to get financial assistance and how to do them.

- Some states have what are called "charity care laws." They require hospitals to provide free or discounted care to patients who meet their eligibility requirements. California, Connecticut, Illinois, Maine, Maryland, Nevada, New Jersey, New York, Rhode Island, and Washington have protections that apply to all hospitals. Louisiana, Oregon, and Texas have protections that apply only to nonprofit or state hospitals. Colorado, Massachusetts, and South Carolina have state-run financial assistance programs.

- It is also possible to negotiate with the hospital *before* you have a procedure or treatment. For example, you can ask for the rate that people with insurance get (it is lower), and sometimes you get a discount for paying up front or promptly. They may also set up a payment plan. Any payment plan should specify that you pay no interest on the debt and that no debt collectors are involved.

- Here's an important tip: at many institutions you shouldn't pay for a hospital bill with a credit card until *after* you have established a payment plan with your healthcare provider. That's because at some hospitals, once you've paid with a credit card it becomes harder, if not impossible, to set up a payment plan.

3. Insurance Plans Don't Cover Certain Medications
Drug costs are a big part of the cost of healthcare, so insurers limit what they will pay for. They do this by establishing a formulary that

has different tiers—from full coverage (many generics and well-accepted medications) to not so much or not at all. There is a process for exceptions based on medical necessity.

Every health insurance plan publishes their formulary with a list of brand-name and generic prescription drugs they cover and their reimbursement rate. They may revise this occasionally during the year or, more usually, annually—so you may have a medication that was covered last year but is not covered this year. It can be shocking.

Why Can't I Get the Brand-Name Medication My Doctor Thinks I Need?
The short answer is that you can, but you may have to pay extra for it—sometimes an unaffordable amount. In most cases there are generic versions of brand-name drugs, and the generic drugs are much cheaper. Usually your doctor will prefer the generics, knowing they are identical to the brand-name drugs. Often your pharmacy will (or in some states will be required to) fill your prescription with the generic version of the same drug even if your doctor prescribes the name brand.

In some cases, a brand-name newer drug still under patent will have a superior therapeutic effect compared to an existing generic drug that is similar but not identical. You may be required by your insurance to take the cheaper generic drug, and they will only pay for the brand-name drug once it's been determined that your response to the first drug is inadequate. Frustrating, right? Yes, but somewhat explainable. The cost of healthcare is very high, and we all benefit if we can get the same or better treatment at lower cost. If we're going to get there, collectively it will require lower-cost treatments, including drugs. But we don't get treated for diseases collectively; we get treated individually. So what can you do to get the preferred medication if you think the generic or older drug isn't right for you?

- Ask your physician's office to contact the insurance company to explain why you need the newer medication. Sometimes the physician needs to receive a prior authorization from the insurance company to prescribe a new or expensive drug. The physician's office might not know this, and you simply experience it as "I can't get my medication." If the doctor receives the prior authorization, the prescription can be filled by your pharmacy.

- Ask your physician's office to determine if there are other administrative hassles. For example, a prescription can be rejected because it was "refilled too soon" or was sent to an out-of-network pharmacy. These problems can usually be resolved between the physician's office and the pharmacy or by sending the prescription to a different pharmacy.

- Call the insurance company yourself to ask for the new medication.

- Sometimes, despite your efforts, the insurance company will insist that you try the generic medication before they will pay for the brand-name drug. If you've exhausted other alternatives and you are determined, negotiate a specific period of time for which you will take the generic treatment before seeking a change. We know of someone who takes medications for a mental health condition and has walked this path repeatedly. They have found that the caseworkers for the insurance company are generally reasonable, so this person has been able to start on a generic medication and then, if the results are not optimal, get switched to the brand-name drug. Yes, it's a hassle, but it often works.

What Can I Do to Reduce the Cost of My Medications?

Drugs can be expensive, and even when the drug you're taking is on your insurer's formulary, your co-pays can be significant. Fortunately, there are some ways that you may be able to lower the cost of your medications.

- If your insurance doesn't cover the medication, or if your out-of-pocket cost is too much to afford, ask your doctor if there is an alternative drug that your insurance covers—either a generic version of the medication or another drug that is known to be effective. You can also ask if the doctor has samples in the office that you can have.
- If your insurance does not cover your medication at all, you can ask for an exception. Your doctor will need to document why you must have the medication. (As noted above, the insurance company may require you to try an alternative medication first, and then if that fails to do the trick, they might consider paying for the one originally prescribed.)
- If your request for an exception is denied, you can file an appeal. This is a smart move, since appeals often succeed. To figure out how to file an appeal, check out the Patient Advocate Foundation (https://www.patientadvocate.org/). If you are on Medicare Part D (the part that covers medication), you can

check the Centers for Medicare and Medicaid Services website, CMS.gov, for assistance or try other resources such as the National Council on Aging (www.ncoa.org/).

- If that fails, there is one more recourse: you can ask for an independent review through your state's insurance regulator. It can take around forty-five days to get the verdict, and there may be a small fee.

- Perhaps before taking on the hassle of dealing with your insurance company, you can look into pharmaceutical company programs designed to make the medication more affordable. Also, companies like GoodRx (www.goodrx.com /prescription/coupons), WellRx (Wellrx.com), and SingleCare (www.singlecare.com/prescriptions/coupons) may offer coupons and discounts. Some charitable organizations can help cover medication costs. Check out the Patient Access Network Foundation (https://www.panfoundation.org) and the National Council on Aging's Benefits Checkup (https://benefitscheckup .org/#/prescreen) online.

4. New Therapies That May Be Lifesaving Can Be Difficult to Get

New and exciting therapies are first made available through clinical trials, in which you may receive the new treatment under closely supervised conditions.

All privately and publicly funded trials around the world are cataloged comprehensively by the National Library of Medicine at the website www.clinicaltrials.gov. In summer 2023, as we were finishing this book, the database included 453,636 research studies in fifty states and almost all the countries in the world. Many of these clinical trials are for medications, but they also include things like medical devices or medical procedures.

How Can I Learn About and Join a Clinical Trial?

In Chapter 6, when we described the creation of your care team, we suggested that you consider which providers and hospitals near you might provide access to a clinical trial suitable to your condition. Regardless of where you end up receiving care, if you or your doctor find a clinical trial that may be right for you, consider being included in the program.

What you can do to find a clinical trial that may help you:

- Ask your doctor. Typically, a doctor and their team will know about many or most of the clinical trials in their department and about some of the other trials in their institution. But doctors won't necessarily know about clinical trials going on in other institutions, even within their own specialty. There are simply too many to keep track of.

- Do your own research, but be aware of two things. First, the language describing clinical trials is complex and technical. It can be very hard for even the most dedicated reader to parse. If you find something interesting, ask your doctor. Even if there is a trial that looks perfectly tailored to your condition, you may not be eligible. The sponsors of clinical trials are looking for very specific participants. You need to have a particular diagnosis, and you may be excluded because of some other condition you have or some other drug you've taken or based on the stage of your treatment.

- Beware of the search for a silver bullet. We've all read about trials that seem to promise miraculous results; they may apply to some folks but not to you. The summer after Cris's second surgery there was a well-publicized trial concerning patients with stage 3 rectal cancer, exactly what Cris had, who had complete remission of cancer without receiving any chemo, radiation, or surgery, just through taking a new drug. Amazing news for those patients, but unavailable for Cris's future use, because it treated a genetic variation in the tumor that Cris didn't have.

How Can I Obtain an Experimental Treatment?

You may also be thinking you should receive a truly experimental treatment outside a clinical trial. Most drug companies are reluctant or outright refuse to make available any drug they are developing before an FDA-controlled phase 3 clinical trial has been completed and they know that it is safe and effective. However, there are situations in which patients can obtain an experimental (not yet approved) treatment—it just takes a concerted effort by their doctor.

However, this can be a complicated and long process. It is not intended to prevent you from accessing lifesaving treatment; rather, the intent is to protect you from dangerous experimentation.

What you can do to access experimental treatment/medication:

- The primary way is to enroll in a clinical trial for that drug or procedure. Information on trials that are recruiting participants is available online from related foundations and healthcare organizations and through clinicaltrials.gov.

- If you don't qualify for an available clinical trial for a specific medication because of your health, your age, or other disqualifying factors and you have tried all approved treatment options, the Right to Try Act may offer a solution. Expanded access—also known as compassionate care—is another way to obtain permission to receive an experimental drug. It is available through the FDA for anyone who has a life-threatening illness for which no standard treatments are available and who is not eligible for a clinical trial. Your physician will need to contact the drug manufacturer and request access for you. If the company agrees to supply the drug, the doctor then applies to the FDA. Information on how to do that is available at FDA.gov under "Expanded Access: Information for Physicians."

5. *Local Hospitals Charge Different Amounts for the Same Services*

You might not be aware that different clinics and hospitals charge different prices for the same treatments—but they do. And sometimes that can affect what you have to pay out-of-pocket, even with good insurance.

One reason that happens is that different healthcare organizations and/or facilities are rated differently by the Centers for Medicaid and Medicare Services (CMS). The higher an organization's rating, the higher their reimbursement rate. A hospital with a four-star rating will receive less health plan reimbursement than a hospital with a five-star rating. So the hospital with the four-star rating may have to charge you more for the same service than a well-compensated hospital does. This may also affect private insurance companies' negotiations with healthcare facilities.

On the other hand, highly rated hospitals may also have the most innovative treatments, cutting-edge technology, and expert medical practitioners—and that's pricey stuff. Even if they receive the highest levels of reimbursement, they may charge the highest prices to cover their expenses.

How Can I Get the Best Treatment for the Best Price?

Since January 2022, the Hospital Transparency Act has required hospitals to provide clear, accessible pricing information online about the items and services they offer. The regulation requires hospitals to share the following:

- Gross charges (as found in the hospital chargemaster, which is the list of all individual items and services offered by a hospital for which the hospital has established a charge, absent any discounts)
- Discounted cash prices (the charge that applies to an individual who pays cash or cash equivalent for a hospital item or service)
- Charges negotiated between the hospital and third-party payers

What you can do to compare hospital pricing and costs:

- If you are having a nonemergency surgery, you can call hospitals and request specific pricing information.
- Make sure to share details on your insurance or lack thereof.
- Share names of any doctors you know you will be working with.
- If you find that the facility where you want to go is more expensive than another, ask about their various programs for providing financial support, discounts, or payment plans.

We can't close out this section on healthcare's big issues without acknowl-edging that many people don't have the luxury of choosing where they get their care or who their doctors are. According to recent research by GoodRx, 80 percent of US counties, containing slightly more than one-third of Americans, lack access to six key healthcare services: (1) pharmacies, (2) primary care providers, (3) hospitals, (4) hospital beds, (5) trauma centers, and (6) low-cost health centers.* And a 2018 Pew Research study concluded that 18 percent of Americans live more than 10 miles away from the nearest hospital. That research also found that 23 percent of people in rural areas say access to good doctors and hospitals is a major problem in their community.† They don't have a choice about where to go unless they are willing to leave their home territory completely. And in rural America the distances that might have to be traveled can be measured in hundreds of miles for the most complex procedures, like transplants or advanced cancer therapies. Finally, people in rural areas are less likely to have health insurance and are more likely to encounter lower-quality care than their urban counterparts, according to a Harvard Medical School study.‡ Those researchers concluded that about 46 million people, or 15

---

* Amanda Nguyen, "Mapping Healthcare Deserts: 80% of the Country Lacks Adequate Access to Healthcare," GoodRx Health, September, 9, 2021, https://www.goodrx.com/healthcare-access/research/healthcare-deserts-80-percent-of-country-lacks-adequate-healthcare-access.
† Onyi Lam, Brian Broderick, and Skye Toor, "How Far Americans Live from the Closest Hospital Differs by Community Type," Pew Research Center, December 12, 2018, https://www.pewresearch.org/short-reads/2018/12/12/how-far-americans-live-from-the-closest-hospital-differs-by-community-type/.
‡ Jacqueline Mitchell, "The Importance of Access," Harvard Medical School, https://hms.harvard.edu/news/importance-access.

percent of the population, are more likely to die of cancer, respiratory diseases, and cardiovascular diseases than those in urban areas.

This challenge also exists in urban areas. A *Pittsburgh Post-Gazette/ Milwaukee Journal* analysis of data from the largest US metropolitan areas shows that "people in poor neighborhoods are less healthy than their more affluent neighbors, but more likely to live in areas with physician shortages and closed hospitals."* The number of hospitals in major cities has fallen by about half since the peak in the 1970s.

We who work in the field are trying to fix healthcare—to make it more affordable and accessible—but challenges remain. For everyone trying to get optimal care without financial burdens, we simply say (once again), stick up for yourself, ask a million questions, rely on your village to help you resolve your questions, and don't be afraid to poke.

Finding the Path to a Good Outcome Despite Endless Obstacles

Mark, a senior executive in a financial services firm, has experienced almost every big issue and annoying thing that can happen to a person entangled in the healthcare system. But it is his resolve and astounding outcomes that make his story so compelling.

Mark: My hearing loss began in 2005, but I dismissed it until 2008, when I admitted I had to get it checked. Over the next two years I saw

---

* Lillian Thomas, "Hospitals, Doctors, Moving Out of Poor City Neighborhoods to More Affluent Areas," *Journal Sentinel,* June 14, 2014, https://archive.jsonline.com/news/health/hospitals-doctors-moving-out-of -poor-city-neighborhoods-to-more-affluent-areas-b99284882z1–262899701 .html/.

eight doctors and was told it was caused by flying too much, eating too many soy products, because I had a deviated septum (I got the operation). Nothing made any difference. Finally I went to a doctor who said he couldn't do anything but I should have an MRI. After twenty doctor's visits, I found out I had a brain tumor.

I wanted to get good treatment, so I pulled some strings and called the chairman of neurosurgery at a major medical system. I got a call back, but he said, "I can't see you for six months and once I do, I probably can't schedule your surgery for three months after that."

The next institution I called said they could take me for surgery sooner, but they wouldn't tell me who the surgeon would be until I got there. I hung up on them. That was not the intake I was looking for.

Then the next day I went to a New York City healthcare system. The doctor who would be the lead physician grew up in my hometown and we were adversaries in sports—but we got over that.

That was May 3, and the surgery was scheduled for June 9. I was out of the hospital by the 11th, alone in a rented apartment in a city that I didn't live in. By my tenth day out, the steroids I was on had made me forty pounds heavier and my head wouldn't stop dripping.

This started a process that culminated in super-antibiotic treatment that they messed up. And to top it off, from the medication, I developed a skin rash. Ultimately, the infection was so bad the doctors had to take the metal plate out that they put in my head after surgery.

I selected one of the best hospitals in the country, but for several weeks, the team failed to prescribe proper meds for the hospital-based infection and didn't discontinue them when they should have. Years later I am still living with facial paralysis due to damage to the facial nerve, which was close to the tumor. I have what I call a bitchy resting face—it's OK, but if I smile it looks like Bell's palsy. So you know what the neurosurgeon said? "Don't smile."

One positive result from all the disasters: I became more emboldened to stick up for myself. When I was trying to get an appointment with a dermatologist, they said they could see me in six weeks. So the next day I called back and said, "I am Dr. Spradley and I have a rash," and they said, "What time can you get here?" It shouldn't be like that, but it is.

As I see it, there are definitely lessons to be learned here. Healthcare needs to progress and improve. Disparities in healthcare for different demographic and racial groups have to be addressed. Everyone needs equal access and care. But it may be improving. It's my belief that in the United States the healthcare system is going through disruptive innovation from technology. We are ushering in the era of precision health, which reimagines medicine so that it focuses on predicting, preventing, and curing disease precisely. And it does that by marrying two seemingly different approaches—high-tech and high-touch. Ultimately, such changes will replace the people I am complaining about, and the services and alliances will improve over time.

And me? How am I? I don't drive anymore because of single-sided deafness and depth-perception problems that make it difficult to interpret relative distances between objects, but I do have two doctorates.

Four Annoying Things: What They Are and How to Handle Them

1. Hospitals Cannot Provide a Good Night's Sleep

It's true that hospitals are notorious for having patients take meds and get blood draws at all hours, and for having alarms ringing in your room, and for loud conversations and bright lights at 3 a.m. But it has gotten much better in many places, since there is widespread recognition of the harm that sleep disturbances can do to a patient's health and healing process. A 2013 study published in *JAMA Internal Medicine* found that about half of patients who are awakened in the middle of the night don't really need to be disturbed—the procedures could be done later, after, say, 7 a.m. It also helps that in 2010 Medicare payments were made contingent in part on patient approval scores, and those scores are specifically related to things like sleep disturbances.

You may be seriously ill and require frequent monitoring—and in that case you probably cannot and do not want to change the pattern of frequent and intrusive monitoring. However, in many situations you can request the following to help you get a good night's sleep:

- Ask your doctor to make sure your medication schedule is as sleep-friendly as possible. Ask for medications that may disturb your sleep to be given during the day.
- Discuss the need for the doctor to have blood test results first thing in the morning (that's why they draw blood during the night). It may be as medically safe to get results later in the morning.
- If your sleep is disturbed by noises outside the room, ask to have your door closed, request earplugs, wear an eye mask, and talk to the nurses and ask them to connect you with the charge nurse. Sometimes people are just oblivious to the fact that they are creating noise. They've been working the night shift so long that 3 a.m. is the middle of their afternoon and a loud conversation with a colleague just seems natural. The nursing

staff should be responsive to your requests. If they aren't, then reach out to the patient advocate or ombudsman that most hospitals have to see what can be done. Or give this job to a village member. You may not like to be a bother, but your village member can be a firm and even fierce advocate on your behalf without hesitation.

- If you are in a double-occupancy room and have a problematic roommate (or their village is a problem), talk with your roommate or discuss the situation with the nurses and your doctor and see what can be done. A transfer to a private room may be possible if one is available, and it may be worth it to pay extra in order to get some peace and rest.

2. Hospital Food Is Terrible

In the past, hospitals turned out the kind of cafeteria food that is the lowest common denominator in terms of freshness and even, surprisingly, nutrition. That too is undergoing a revolution. But it is still difficult to get fed when you're hungry (dinner can show up at 4:30 p.m.) or reliably get the kind of food you can or want to eat. And food is chosen and prepared to avoid side effects for everyone. So for many palates, that means bland, unsalted, unseasoned meals. Distressingly, you can still find fast-food outlets in many hospitals, though they are disappearing. Even though you might despair at the lack of a tasty meal, don't give in and eat highly processed, nutrition-lacking foods that certainly won't make you feel better and might make you feel worse.

Hospitals can accommodate vegetarians, vegans, people with religious food restrictions, and those who have food allergies or intolerances.

You might opt for one of those choices, as the food may be somewhat more carefully prepared. But if you're getting the regular meal service, you can still establish some ground rules.

- Your doctor can order a cardiac diet for you (controlled fat content) or a low-carb diet, for example, which may improve the quality of what you get.
- Ask your doctor if there are foods you should avoid.
- Whenever there is a menu to choose from, choose wisely. It's increasingly rare that the food service serves a standard meal to everyone, but if that's what's offered, be clear about which foods you do not want to receive. It's a start.
- Consider asking your village to take responsibility for bringing you healthy, tasty food once a day. That may be a good solution, but be careful that you don't eat things you shouldn't.

3. Half the Time I Don't Even Know the Name of the Doctor Who Came to Examine Me

Your surgeon, specialist, or primary care physician has many patients to see each day and may stop in first thing in the morning to check up on you—but after that colleagues and residents who work with the doctor are likely to pop in, review your chart, and make sure all is going well. If you're groggy or distracted, they can come and go before you have a chance to figure out who they are or what they're doing. In good hospitals with strong patient experience practices, everyone coming in the room will identify themselves to you. But that's not the practice everywhere.

If you have members of your village in the room with you, they can help you keep track of the clinicians you see. It's asking a lot of yourself, post-surgery or post-procedure, to ask each clinician their name, if they're a doctor or some other kind of clinician, what their field of specialization is, and why they are examining you or checking on you.

Later, when you are more focused and feeling up to it, if the clinicians visiting your room don't introduce themselves upon entering and say why they are visiting (and you don't know who they are or what they do), you can ask them the following questions. (Also, share this list with your village members so that they can get detailed info more easily.)

- What is your name, your role in my care, and your area of specialization?
- Who is your supervising physician or colleague? What brings you here today?
- Has something changed about my condition, or is there anything I should know? What is it that you are looking for or interested in evaluating about my condition?
- I have some questions. Should I ask you, or wait for the physician who is managing my care?

4. In This Digital Age You Still Have to Fill Out Endless Forms and Questionnaires with Identical Information

Healthcare institutions are trying to streamline the information-collecting process, and this problem is slowly going away. There are nationwide networks that now allow doctors and hospitals to share digital healthcare records with the patient's consent. Nearly 90 percent of all hospitals and clinics in the United States are connected to one of these networks for patients, making it much easier for doctors to know a patient's in-depth medical history no matter where they live or where they received care.

But sometimes the left hand still doesn't have access to what the right hand is doing, and you are too often asked to provide the same information repeatedly. And there are still some requirements from government agencies and businesses for paper records and faxes that have not yet been eliminated from healthcare.

So how can you skip filling out endless forms and questionnaires? To start, ask your providers if they can get records from your previous care. Beyond that, sorry, for this one we have no answer. You've got to give them the information they need when and how they need it. Just breathe deeply and be thankful for the care you are going to insist you receive. And don't yell at the desk receptionist, the doctor, or the nurse. You can yell at your local hospital CIO. Tell them Ed and Cris sent you.

We know this doesn't address all the wrongheaded or frustrating things that come up when you are in the hospital, but we hope it helps sort out some of the most bewildering and irritating issues—and makes you (and your village) feel empowered to tackle them head-on and come out on top.

Nine

The Art of Caregiving

The rewards and challenges

In every village there are one or two people who are the true caregivers, the people who are with the patient the most, through the hardest parts of the journey. If you are a caregiver, not just a run-of-the-mill village member, this chapter is for you.

Caregivers are the lifeline of every patient. They help translate what doctors say, remember the right questions to ask, make sure medical care is delivered in a timely way, drive to appointments, and see to it that the patient—a.k.a. their loved one—is fed and clothed, takes the right meds at the right time, and knows that they are not alone. It could wear you out just to read that sentence, let alone live it day in and day out.

We were blessed with supportive and loving caregivers, but that doesn't mean they weren't frustrated by our actions or inactions, exhausted by the physical and mental strain of caring, and desperate to have a break now and then—even if they didn't want to admit it to themselves or to us!

And having watched them as they took care of us, we have learned just how important it is for caregivers to care for themselves and to have access to advice and support from experts in the field—and other caregivers.

So, we're going to let our caregivers and caregiving experts show you how you can deliver the best care to your loved one—and yourself.

We'll add our two cents by letting you know what we thought was most beneficial—and most irritating—about being on the receiving end of all that care and fuss and bother (because that is what it seems like sometimes).

A Digital Village for Patients and Caregivers

Caring Bridge is a nonprofit dedicated to helping people through their health journeys. Its vision is that no patient should go through a health journey alone. CaringBridge lets every patient and/or caretaker create their own site on which to share information about a patient's journey and needs—and the caretaker's needs as well. More than 300,000 people use the ad-free, not-for-profit platform every day, sharing health updates and rallying around loved ones. Every ten minutes there's a new CaringBridge site made to share updates and get support. And every hour, 1,800 messages of encouragement are shared on a loved one's site. Increasingly, CaringBridge has come to understand that while its website and app are about a patient's journey, they're also about the journey of the caregiver and for addressing the sense of loneliness that can occur from the intense job of caregiving.

Cris is on the board and says, "It's been a remarkable source of information and support for me, personally—I had my own site—and for millions of others. The online tools and resources are effective in helping patients and their caregivers get through a health journey."

There are many resources for caregivers on the CaringBridge website (https://admin.caringbridge.org/resources/tips-for-caregivers/). One example of a popular article is "10 Important Tips for Caregivers, from Caregivers." They are:

1. Learn to communicate effectively (both with your loved one and the medical team).
2. Take care of *you*.
3. Acknowledge your loved one's limitations.
4. Accept help from your community, family, and friends.
5. Be realistic.
6. Learn how to provide proper physical care.
7. Be open to new methods of care.
8. Stay connected with the outside world.
9. Get organized.
10. Start a CaringBridge site.

Tips for Caregivers

In addition to the great advice available from caregiver support organizations like CaringBridge, our experiences lead us to suggest eight additional tips for caregivers.

Communicate with Medical Professionals

Don't be afraid to ask questions throughout the treatment and after—if necessary, over and over! And don't let them dismiss your or your loved one's concerns.

Also, help out the doctors by trying to make sure that your loved one doesn't clam up around them. Help the patient admit to themselves, and then to their doctors, how they are feeling, what their symptoms are, and what they are worried about. Being stoic isn't to the patient's advantage when you are with the doctors.

Finally, there are some things you may need to ask the doctor, perhaps out of earshot of your loved one: "How is my loved one doing, really?" "What can I expect?" "What will they need from me?"

Ask Questions and Take Notes

Ask as many questions as you need (write them down ahead of time if you know what they are), and write down the doctor's responses in as much detail as you need to. If something isn't clear to you or your loved one, ask the medical professionals to explain it differently or more thoroughly. Your loved one will most likely not be able to hear or retain all the details that are shared in an appointment—anxiety can interfere with clear cognition.

But equally important, while you want to stay connected with your patient, you also want to make sure the patient is in charge, not you. They get to choose how they want to pursue this journey. Don't interfere with that by being pushier than they want or meeker than they need.

Develop a System for Long-Distance Caregiving

Maybe you have an aging parent who lives a few hours away. Or maybe one of your children, who lives out of state, has recently suffered an injury. You want to care for them, but you are not able to be there at all—or only intermittently. That calls for some creative use of technology so that you can communicate well with the person you are caring for, including while participating in appointments and helping with medical decisions when appropriate.

- Make sure you and the patient have the appropriate technology that you both know how to use—or find someone close to your loved one who can help. (During Cris's second cancer experience, one of his daughters started up an Apple FaceTime call on Cris's phone so that his oncologist could answer his and his daughter's questions.)

- Either you and/or your loved one need to make sure you have medical information you might need to share with the doctor(s) on the call. The doctors caring for your loved one should have the medical information availiable, but if you are coordinating between health systems you may need to share information between providers.

- Before calls with doctors, take time to talk with your loved one and develop a list of questions that you want to ask. Write them down.

Caregiving at a distance is more than just about medical facts and appointments with doctors. But that communication is critical for your loved one. Be the best medical secretary and advocate you possibly can be.

Be There to Listen

As a caregiver, you may want to try to fix a situation right away. But sometimes that's not what a patient needs or wants. Instead, they may simply need an empathetic ear to listen to them. You should validate the patient's thoughts and feelings and help them learn to process their emotions. At least initially, hold off on giving advice or suggestions. This will create a safe environment for the patient to speak openly and unload what they're feeling. When they want advice or an opinion, they'll ask for it.

Give Your Loved One Space When They Need It

There are going to be days and even weeks when a patient will depend on you. You'll help them with meals, ensure they take their medication on time, run errands on their behalf, interface with doctors. As a caregiver, it's completely normal to unconsciously develop a mindset that the patient needs you every second of the day—but it's not always true.

As time passes, consider giving your loved one some space and independence. They're likely frustrated already about having much of their autonomy taken away. If there are things they can and *want* to do on their own, allow them to have that opportunity. Plus, it gives you a break.

Embrace Any Emotions You Feel

Being a caregiver can be incredibly challenging. Not only are you taking on a lot of responsibility, but you're also taking care of someone who might feel a lot of negative, disheartening emotions. Eventually these emotions can get to you.

It's best not to keep things bottled up. Allow yourself to feel and process. Whether you need to cry, pray, or take a time-out, permit yourself to do so.

Some days will be good, and some days will be bad. Whatever you're experiencing, give yourself the same grace you'd give to others. Take it one moment at a time, and be gentle with yourself.

Sometimes journaling can help with working through the overwhelming amount of emotions you may feel. Consider using a notebook to write down your thoughts or questions as they arise. You can make bullet lists of positive affirmations, or even reread old entries to find power and strength.

Research shows that caregiving takes a mental and physical toll. For example, a 2021 study, "Association Between Children with Life-Threatening Conditions and Their Parents' and Siblings' Mental and Physical Health," published in *JAMA Network Open*, found that mothers, fathers, sisters, and brothers of children with serious illness had higher overall rates of healthcare encounters, diagnoses, and prescriptions than in families not contending with that challenge.

Join a Support Group for Caregivers

Even if you have the support of family and friends, they may not totally understand what you're going through. That's where caregiver support groups can be incredibly helpful.

These support groups are filled with people going through similar situations as you. Whether these groups are in-person or online, you'll find people who can empathize with all the challenges and emotions you're going through.

Vent about your frustration, receive words of encouragement, and even get advice and recommendations. You'll also have the opportunity to inspire and help others by sharing your story. Check out Family Caregiver Alliance (https://www.caregiver.org/) for information on online groups as well as a state-by-state inventory of caregiver-support programs.

Reach Out to Friends and Family for Support

Even though you might be excellent at giving help, it can be difficult to receive it. When it comes to caregiving, try to get in the mindset that you deserve support as well. Also be aware that often people want to lend a hand, but they may not know how. It's important to bring them into the fold so that they're there when you need them most.

The Bottom Line

When someone who is near and dear to you is in the hospital with an acute illness or at home contending with a long-term chronic illness, it may feel downright selfish to worry about how you are doing and how your health is. But it is not. You do no favors for a patient by neglecting your own health or allowing yourself to become weary, anxious, short-tempered, or resentful. That can happen when you are caregiving—it's only human and nothing to be ashamed of. It's simply a signal that you need to step back, breathe, and figure out how to optimize the care you give while still looking out for your well-being. Put on your own oxygen mask before assisting others.

That's the short form—now let's dive in with some real-life caregivers' stories and a more detailed look at how you can master the art of caregiving.

Caring for Cris

You could say that the name Cris is a short form of the word *crisis*. His caretakers report he did everything he could to make his very serious health journey seem like less of a crisis.

> *From his daughter Emily: The first time he told me he was sick, he very calmly said, "We need to talk about something." He was so calm it almost didn't sink in until later the same night. Because he downplayed it so much, I had a delayed reaction. Later, it was clear, he was thinking about me, not himself.*

Cris's diagnosis and treatment coincided with Emily coming back to the United States from studying in Europe and graduating from college. She moved in with him and juggled finding a job, starting her new life, and providing the care her dad needed and wanted.

Emily: Dad says I did so much, but I thought I did the bare minimum. After all, he's my dad, and I'm going to take care of him!

What I did felt natural to do, just helping out. But after a while it all kind of added up. Once I got a job, there were times I would go to work and not be around cancer, and it made me realize I was spending a lot of time worrying about my dad as he went through intense chemo. He would decline and then get better and then dive-bomb into chemo again. At work, being with folks who were healthy kind of made me wish I wasn't living that reality.

When he relapsed . . . I was very, very afraid. I took a week and went to see my mom in California. I just needed to be away from cancer for a little bit. I talked to dad every day, but I was living a life where I wasn't a cancer caretaker. More than I knew, it had taken a toll on me.

I want to tell other caretakers, do not lose your own separate life and friends and existence outside of caretaking. When I had a moment outside of cancer I could come back and be even more caring and helpful. It was hard to leave, and I timed it so I was gone when he had finished chemo and hadn't started radiation yet, but it was important to do—for me and for Dad.

Cris's girlfriend, Anne-Marie, lives in Rochester, where she is an M.D. radiologist at Mayo Clinic, ninety minutes away from Cris and Emily in St. Paul. Emily says the two of them meshed gracefully as caretakers.

Anne-Marie juggled two worlds—and two different coping styles, hers and Cris's—while caring for him. She was a doctor, working with her colleagues to do imaging that would provide a diagnosis (often a tough one) to patients, and she was a loved one, sharing a sometimes frightening, often demanding medical journey with Cris.

> *Anne-Marie: Initially Cris, of course, downplayed his symptoms. They came up fairly suddenly, but he was in enough pain that I knew there was something serious going on. When he called for an appointment, they said it would be a couple of months. I told him to contact the doctor or her nurse directly, which he was aghast about, but he did that and got the ball rolling. He always thinks that the medical team is too busy for him, but he should be thinking that they want to hear from him in a timely manner so that they can take care of things.*

Anne-Marie describes herself as the kind of person who comes across as a bit aloof, but that's just a façade.

> *Anne-Marie: I don't show a lot of emotion in front of other people. It makes people think I don't ever need any help and that I am unfazed by this kind of caretaking. Luckily, I have a wonderfully supportive sister and a couple of girlfriends who are like sisters, and I can be completely honest with them and say the things I would never say to the person I am caring for!*
>
> *I really needed that support, because being the girlfriend (and not for that long when he was first diagnosed) rather than the spouse, I wasn't really a part of Cris's long-term social world yet, so there wasn't really anyone in his world I could turn to.*

Outside of Emily and Hannah, Cris doesn't have a lot of family support either. I do think it's a different family dynamic than mine. He's got amazing friends, and they are his family.

There was a time, after he relapsed, when it was rough going and he was really down. He got to the point where he said, "I can't do this anymore." My answer was, "Yes you can! You are doing it!" I think being a cheerleader helps. At that point, it was good to be tough-minded. But we didn't always mesh.

My bottom line: Caregiving is a tangled mess sometimes! Everyone—patients and caregivers—has a day at the bottom, but no matter how bad you feel, you need to know how you act has an effect. You also have to get able to understand that and to forgive any slights. There's a bigger picture and a longer road you want to travel down together.

Caring for Ed

Simran, Ed's wife, is a nurse (BSN/MSN/DNP) and CEO of Sim's MedSpa. She spent her younger years as a caregiver for her mother, who was completely paralyzed in the last few years of her life. When Ed had a heart attack and then was diagnosed with cancer, she found it to be a much different situation.

Simran: With my mom, I was much younger, and it was a different culture and a different time. She was very demanding and verbally abusive. She'd be throwing things and then apologize later on.

The best part of caring for Ed was that he wasn't very fussy. But men don't like to be sick, and they want to be macho. Ed would constantly say "I'm fine, I'm fine." I would reply, "No, you are not. You are red-faced and in pain. Take your pain medication." But he wouldn't.

I had to accept that you can't force anyone to do anything; you just have to let them live and learn. If you force the issue you take the person's independence away. But at the same time, you want them to get better and to do it by cooperating with the medical advice they get.

It was frustrating, so I'd call my best friend and she'd say, "Take a deep breath. Ask your daughter or son to come take over." Then I could go work out—which helped a lot. Other times I would take him with me, and he would sit and watch as I worked out. That was an outing for us both. We often took short trips to the mall or anywhere to give him a feeling of freedom and to interact with the world. It was a healing thing for him.

I can summarize what I've learned about caregiving this way:

1. *In the hospital you have to be their eyes, ears, and advocate. Even as a member of the Cleveland Clinic staff we had issues when Ed had his prostatectomy. Hours went by, and I couldn't see him in recovery; they didn't have a room ready for him. I had to throw a tantrum to get to see him and to find out what his condition was. It was a lesson in how important it is to have a caregiver in the hospital with you who can ask a million questions about what is being done to the patient, the medications they are prescribed, and the therapy they are—or are not—getting.*

2. *During in-hospital recovery and at home, you want to take care of what your loved one needs—just ask them to tell you what it is. And then be patient. I am outspoken, and sometimes I had to bite my tongue.*

3. *Listen more than talk—hear what they are saying about how they feel and what they need. Remember your loved*

one doesn't want to be sick, and you, the caretaker, are healthy. That alone can cause tension.

4. *Stay on top of the medical team in the hospital—from long distance if you must. When Ed, who is a triathlete, had his heart attack they didn't know his regular heart rate was about 30 to 35 beats a minute. It went down to around 28. Now, that's not the same situation as it might be for someone whose heart rate is usually 75. Until I flew down to South Carolina and was with him in the hospital those kinds of important details were missed.*

5. *You also want to teach independence—not dependency. The first twenty-four hours of a medical crisis you give them everything they need. Then on day three you ask them to walk ten steps or make their own coffee, but be right there to offer support if they run into trouble.*

6. *Respect your patient's need for alone time. You don't want to smother them.*

7. *You don't want to obliterate your life outside of caretaking. In the process of being a caregiver I learned that it was very important for me to have self-care. I told myself, "Put on your makeup and get ready for the day. Don't stay in your PJs. Continue your normal life—don't let your loved one's sickness disrupt that."*

A Difficult Subject: Planning for the Worst

The pressure on caregivers, the anxiety and uncertainty both they and patients feel, the isolation that illness can impose—all of this makes the caregiving relationship a lot to juggle for everyone involved. A particularly important topic, though a difficult one, is to make sure you are on the same page with your spouse or closest loved ones about what their wishes are should they be in a life-threatening or end-of-life situation.

Silvia Perez-Protto, M.D., M.Sc., FCCM, is the medical director of the End of Life Center at Cleveland Clinic, where she developed the Advance Care Planning program. Caretaking, she says, is much easier when patient and caretaker have talked to each other *before* there is a health crisis about their wishes around medical care, family support, caretaking, and end of life.

"When people don't share their wishes, it makes caretaking and end-of-life decisions very hard on the caretakers and family," she says. "Creating documents that outline your wishes and provide legal protection for them—and then talking to your family about those wishes—removes conflict or uncertainty and helps build empathy."

A living will's expressed wishes supersede the decisions of anyone with healthcare power of attorney, if they are in conflict. "I recommend that you review and, if you want, revise the document every ten years," says Dr. Perez-Protto. "And after each review/revision, you need to let your family and close friends know the decisions you have made."

If you need a guide to help you create these documents. there are some good resources:

- The Conversation Project provides information about how to have a conversation with loved ones and how to talk to your doctors. Check out https://theconversationproject.org/.
- Five Wishes offers guidance at https://www.fivewishes.org/.
- Prepare for Your Care, at https://prepareforyourcare.org, has a Spanish-language version.

There is even an organization called Death over Dinner that has hundreds of thousands of past and current participants who follow their guidelines for bringing the family together at the dinner table to discuss healthcare wishes and end-of-life planning.

The Caregiver's Checklist

When you are thrown into the role of caregiver, it is very helpful to identify your potential tasks/duties and write out details and information that can help you feel more confident about fulfilling the demands of your new role.

- Get details of your loved one's medical needs from the doctors.
- Ask about any special caregiving skills you may need to learn and develop. Sometimes you can be trained how to help change dressings, eliminate waste, and so on.
- Start a list that notes all your medications and when they are taken, when meals are eaten, bathroom schedules, et cetera.
- Have a list of all doctors' names and contact info. Have copies of the patient's insurance and other important ID numbers.
- Determine who has the healthcare proxy—or make sure to establish one. Check that there is a living will.
- Write out a list of the patient's needs regarding meals, bathing, medication, bathrooming, and so forth.
- Identify adjustments to the layout and organization of the bedroom at home that will facilitate caring and make your loved one more comfortable.
- With the patient's consent, sign up to have proxy access to the patient's medical records via the online portal or app.

Ed and Cris on Receiving Caregiving

In closing this chapter, we both want to say how deeply we appreciate the patience and perseverance that our loved ones showed us while we were in the hospital and at home recovering.

We both came to realize that our caregivers were often smarter about what we should do and about our needs than we were. The amazing thing is that they let us come to this understanding on our own, so that it stuck with us and changed how we interact even today, when mutual daily caretaking is an expression of everyday love and friendship.

To have made a journey through two bouts of cancer (Cris) and a heart attack and cancer (Ed) and come out the other side, working full speed, laughing frequently, traveling comfortably, and loving more intensely, is a gift from them that we are eternally grateful for. We hope that our deep appreciation in some way softens the hard times and bad behavior that we exhibited while we were actively recovering. And we hope sharing our stories will make the journey that the patient and caregiver are on together less bumpy and maybe even more rewarding.

Afterword

Congratulations—you made it to the end of this book! We know it is hard to take the time to read while you're in the midst of a significant health event. But while we don't get to decide what happens in our lives, we do get to decide how to respond. Hopefully this book gives you some ideas about how you might craft your response.

As the words for this book were painstakingly crafted and recrafted, we were sustained by how much we care about what happens to you. Our motivation has been you and your journey. We would not have invested the time, the energy, and the tears (lots of tears) otherwise. We have bathed the writing in thoughts and prayers.

All of our proceeds from the sale of this book are donated in your honor directly to Mayo Clinic, earmarked to fund cancer research.

Believing in the best for you and your family, may this book be a hand you can hold through your healthcare journey.

—Cris and Ed

Acknowledgments

I am thankful for everyone who gave time to participate in our focus groups. We conducted a few dozen all around the country. I appreciate your inputs, and you will see many of your ideas in these pages. Your willingness to share your ideas will help millions of patients and their families. That is humanity.

Oh, my princess-wife, Simran Marx. The journey of book writing is long and time-consuming. You remained unwavering and even encouraging in your support. I am blessed.

My friend and co-author, Cris. At first, I admired you from a distance and was impressed. I then became a peer, and you taught me things about leadership and strategy. Next, we became friends, and the authenticity I admired from a distance was even more real close-up. In the process of writing this book together I fell in love with the man himself. Closer than a brother. Bonded by cancer. Aligned by purpose.

My dear editor, Kalia Doner. I recall our first meeting, when Cris and I were like, "Hell yes, we need her!" I love your no-nonsense approach, and you taught me how to be a better writer, maybe even a better person. Thank you, Mayo Clinic Press, for your support. Nina Wiener, you have been our cheerleader since the start.

—Ed

My thanks and deepest respect go out to every famous and anonymous contributor to the science and delivery of cures.

And thanks to all the clinicians and supporting staff who cured me twice with uncommon grace and skill.

To the countless people with whom I talked about this book, my sincerest thanks for your contributions, which you will see in these pages.

To my friend and co-author, Ed, who invented this book and drove it to completion through thick and thin, you are a man with a giant heart and a gifted brain who never seems to rest on your triathlon through life. An inspiration. My brother from another mother.

To all my caregivers: Hannah, Emily, Anne-Marie, and my ever-generous friends.

And to Mayo Clinic, Mayo Clinic Press, Nina Wiener and the editorial staff, and the great and gracious Kalia Doner.

—Cris